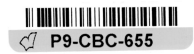
Pharmacy Technician Certification

Quick-Study Guide

Third Edition

Pharmacy Technician Certification

Quick-Study Guide

Third Edition

Susan Moss Marks, BPharm
Educational Services Consultant
Pharmacist and Technician Programs
Phoenix, Arizona

William A. Hopkins, Jr., PharmD, FACA
President
Clinical Pharmacy Consultants of North Georgia
Big Canoe, Georgia

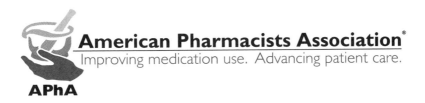

American Pharmacists Association®
Improving medication use. Advancing patient care.
APhA

Washington, D.C.

Acquisitions Editor: Sandra J. Cannon
Managing Editor: Linda L. Young
Proofreader: Eileen Kramer
Compositor: Graphics by Design
Cover Designer: Ruth Schmuff, Plum Creative Associates, LLC; Scott Neitzke, APhA Creative Services

©Copyright 2006 by the American Pharmacists Association
Published by the American Pharmacists Association
1100 15th Street, N.W., Suite 400
Washington, D.C. 20005-1707
www.aphanet.org

APhA was founded in 1852 as the American Pharmaceutical Association

To comment on this book via e-mail, send your message to the publisher at aphanet.org

Library of Congress Cataloging-in-Publication Data

Marks, Susan Moss.
  Pharmacy technician certification : quick-study guide / Susan Moss
Marks, William A. Hopkins, Jr. -- 3rd ed.
      p. ; cm.
  Includes bibliographical references.
  ISBN-13: 978-1-58212-098-0
  ISBN-10: 1-58212-098-6
  1. Pharmacy technicians--Examinations, questions, etc. 2. Pharmacy
technicians--Outlines, syllabi, etc. I. Hopkins, William A. (William
Alexander), 1947- II. Title.
  [DNLM: 1. Pharmacy--Examination Questions. 2. Pharmacy--Outlines. 3.
Pharmacists' Aides--Examination Questions. 4. Pharmacists'
Aides--Outlines. QV 18.2 M346p 2006]

  RS122.95.M37 2006
  615'.1076--dc22

                                                            2006023911

How to Order This Book
By phone: 800-878-0729 (domestic)
Online: www.pharmacist.com
VISA®, MasterCard®, and American Express® cards accepted.

Contents

Section I

Assisting the Pharmacist in Serving Patients

Includes activities related to prescription dispensing and medication distribution, including:

- receiving and processing prescriptions and medication orders
- obtaining and entering information in the patient profile
- collecting data to help the pharmacist monitor patient outcomes
- preparing sterile products

Chapter One

Receiving Prescriptions and Medication Orders

I. Key Terms and Concepts

A. Prescriptions
1. A prescription is an order for the preparation and administration of a drug or nondrug remedy issued by a licensed medical practitioner who is authorized by state law to prescribe. Prescriptions may be presented to the pharmacy in written form or via telephone, fax, or computer, depending on individual state laws. Prescribers may include physicians, dentists, veterinarians, nurse practitioners, and physician assistants. Prescriptions are usually filled in an outpatient pharmacy for use by the patient on an ambulatory basis.

B. Medication orders
1. A medication order, like a prescription, is a written order for the preparation and administration of medication, issued by a licensed medical practitioner who is authorized to prescribe. Medication orders are intended for patients in an inpatient (institutional) setting.

C. Trade/proprietary drug name
1. The terms *trade* and *proprietary* refer to the manufacturer's brand name (protected by trademark) for a particular drug.

D. Generic/nonproprietary drug name
1. The terms *generic* and *nonproprietary* refer to a drug name not protected by a trademark, which is usually descriptive of its chemical structure.

II. Understanding Prescriptions and Medication Orders

A. Prescriptions should contain the following information:
1. Patient information
   a. The prescription order should include the patient's name, age, address, and telephone number.

2. Date
   a. The date the prescriber wrote the prescription order.

3. Name of the product
   a. The drug name may be written as either the generic or trade name.

4. Strength of the product
   a. The strength should always be included to avoid misinterpretation, but may not be included if only one strength is commercially available, or if otherwise inappropriate (e.g., devices). Strength may also be excluded in products that consist of a combination of two or more drugs for which only one drug:drug concentration ratio is commercially available.

5. Dosage form
   a. The dosage form may not be included if only one dosage form is commercially available. See Appendix A for a list of common dosage forms.

6. Quantity of medication to be dispensed
   a. The quantity represents the number of units or dosage forms (e.g., tablets, ounces, grams) to be dispensed. It may not be included if the quantity to be dispensed can be calculated from the physician's directions and duration of therapy (e.g., 3 month supply). May also be written as q.s. *(a sufficient quantity)* or q.s. ad *(a sufficient quantity to make)*.

7. Directions for preparation
   a. Instructions to the pharmacist for compounding or preparing a product may be included. See Appendix B for terminology and abbreviations frequently used for this purpose.

8. Directions for labeling
   a. Prescriber's instructions to the pharmacist on what information should be included on the prescription label.

9. Directions for the patient to be included on the prescription label
   a. Instructions for the patient on how to use the medication properly. Appendix B lists terminology and abbreviations frequently used.
      (1) Route of administration. See Appendix A for a list of drug administration routes.

      (2) Dosage and dosage schedule. The quantity of medication to be taken by the patient and the schedule (frequency and/or time) of administration.

10. Refill information
    a. The prescriber's instructions for the number of refills that may be dispensed from the prescription order. If no information is provided, no refills are authorized. A prescriber may also write "no refills" or "NR" on the prescription order.

11. Prescriber information
    a. Prescriber's name, address, and telephone number

    b. Prescriber's Drug Enforcement Administration (DEA) number

    c. Prescriber's signature (unless the prescription is received by telephone)

B. Medication orders
1. Patient information
    a. While every medication order may not include in-depth patient information (diagnosis, concurrent therapies, etc.), the patient profile should contain this information as transcribed from previous orders. Medication orders typically include the following information:
        (1) Patient's name, birth date, room number, identification number
        (2) Indication for use of the medication (why the drug is being ordered)
        (3) Allergies or other information necessary to process the medication order

2. Date the medication order was written

3. Time of day that the medication order was written
    a. Time is an important factor in the institutional setting where patients are cared for on a 24-hour basis.

4. Name of the product
    a. Generic and/or trade name of the product

5. Strength of the product
    a. The strength should always be included to avoid misinterpretation, but may not be included if only one strength is commercially available, or if otherwise inappropriate (e.g., devices). Strength may also be excluded in products that consist of a combination of two or more drugs for which only one drug:drug concentration ratio is commercially available.

6. Dosage form
    a. The dosage form may not be included if only one dosage form is commercially available. See Appendix A for a list of common dosage forms.

7. Prescriber information
    a. Name and signature of the prescriber. The prescriber is usually the patient's primary physician, but may be another attending physician or resident. The signature of the prescriber is not required when the order is received verbally, either by telephone or through another authorized health care professional. In these cases, the name or initial of the recipient (e.g., attending registered nurse or pharmacist) must be included on the medication order.

8. Directions for preparation
    a. Instructions to the pharmacist for compounding or preparing a product may be included. See Appendix B for terminology and abbreviations frequently used for this purpose.

9. Directions for administration
    a. Instructions for the nurse or other health care provider on how to administer the medication properly.
        (1) Route of administration. See Appendix A for a list of drug administration routes.

        (2) Dosage and dosage schedule. The quantity of medication to be taken and the schedule (frequency and/or time) of administration.

b. Duration of therapy. Instructions describing how long the patient should receive the medication.

c. Other instructions for administration. These may include detailed information on administration and scheduling of the drug such as start date for medication use, tapering dosages, administration times related to laboratory tests, etc.

III. Receiving New Prescriptions and Medication Orders

A. Accepting new prescriptions/medication orders from patient/patient's representative, prescriber, or other health care professionals. Performing this function requires the technician to be knowledgeable about the information required on prescriptions and medication orders.
   1. Written orders
      a. Ambulatory/outpatient setting
         (1) Prescriptions may be presented to the pharmacy in various ways. In the outpatient setting, new prescriptions are typically brought to the pharmacy by the patient or patient's representative. Depending on state laws, the prescriber may also send written prescription orders via fax.

      b. Institutional/inpatient setting
         (1) In the institutional setting, a written medication order may be presented to the pharmacy department by a physician, nurse, other health care professional or messenger; transmitted electronically through an in-house computer system; or sent to the pharmacy via a pneumatic tube system.

   2. Electronic prescriptions/medication orders
      a. Fax and computer-generated prescriptions/medication orders
         (1) Fax and computer-generated orders are electronic versions of written orders and should be received and processed in the same manner.

   3. Telephone orders
      a. Verbal orders for medications (whether received by telephone or in person) may be accepted only by a licensed pharmacist or, in some states, by a supervised pharmacy intern. In the institutional setting, a registered nurse may also receive and transcribe telephone orders from the prescriber.

IV. Receiving Prescription Refill and Transfer Requests

A. Accepting refill requests from patient/patient's representative or prescriber
   1. Receiving refill requests requires the technician to be knowledgeable about what information is required to process refills and how to obtain appropriate authorization for refills if necessary.

B. Accepting refill requests electronically
   1. Telephone orders
      a. The following information should be obtained when receiving oral requests for refills from patients, patients' representatives, or prescribers:

      (1) Patient's name and telephone number

      (2) Prescription number

      (3) Drug name, strength, and quantity

      (4) Prescriber information

      (5) Reimbursement mechanisms/third-party-payer information

  2. Fax and computer-generated refill requests
     a. The information listed above also should be included in fax requests for refills. The prescriber must be contacted if more information is needed.

C. Contacting prescribers for clarification/authorization of prescription or medication order refills
  1. At the direction of the supervising pharmacist, technicians may be responsible for calling prescribers to obtain authorization for prescription refills or to renew medication orders that have expired. The following information should be provided to the prescriber or the prescriber's representative:
     a. Pharmacy's name and telephone number

     b. Patient's name

     c. Drug name, strength, and quantity

     d. Date of last refill

     e. Prescription directions

     f. Description of information that needs to be clarified, confirmed, or authorized

D. Transferring and accepting transfers of prescriptions or medication orders
  1. At the direction of the supervising pharmacist, technicians may be responsible for transferring prescriptions to another pharmacy or receiving prescriptions transferred by another pharmacy. The following information should be provided to the pharmacy receiving the transfer, and requested by the technician or pharmacist accepting a transferred prescription:
     a. Pharmacy's name and telephone number

     b. Patient's name and telephone number

     c. Drug name, strength, quantity, and instructions for use

     d. Date of original prescription

     e. Date of last refill

f. Physician's name and telephone number

g. Name of technician and/or pharmacist sending and receiving the transferred prescription

h. Original prescription number

V. Assessing Prescriptions and Medication Orders

A. Assessing the prescription or medication order for accuracy and completeness requires the technician to understand the information being presented and to ask appropriate questions when necessary. Evaluating the prescription or medication order should include checking the accuracy and completeness of the following:

1. Patient information. Using the criteria described above, ascertain that appropriate patient information is included on the prescription/medication order.
   a. Prescriptions
      (1) Patient's name, age, address, known allergies

   b. Medication orders
      (1) Patient's name, birth date, room number, identification number, allergies, indications, and any other pertinent information necessary for processing the medication order. Other relevant patient information (e.g., diagnosis) may be verified by checking the patient profile.

2. Drug and product availability
   a. Verify that the product or drug name, strength, and dosage form are written in a manner consistent with commercially available products. This requires knowledge of available products, prescription medications, dosage forms, strengths, etc.

3. Authenticity
   a. Assess whether the prescription/medication order appears to be legitimate (e.g., prescriber's signature is authentic).

4. Legality
   a. Assess whether the prescription/medication order is legal. This includes verifying that the order is in compliance with federal and state laws, etc.

5. Reimbursement eligibility
   a. Determine whether the patient is covered by the appropriate insurance or third-party payer and that the drug (and the quantity of drug prescribed) is eligible for reimbursement according to the payer's policies. Confirm that the pharmacy accepts the patient's insurance carrier.

   b. Assist the patient or the patient's representative in choosing the best payment assistance plan if multiple plans are available to the patient.

VI. Chapter Summary

A. As front-line health care practitioners, pharmacy technicians must understand all aspects of receiving prescriptions and medication orders.

B. Technicians should be familiar with information required on prescriptions and medication orders. They must also know how to accept new orders, refill requests and transfers from health care professionals, and be able to assess orders for clarity, completeness, accuracy, authenticity, and legality.

VII. Questions for Discussion

A. Discuss various differences between prescription orders and medication orders (information requirements, intent, quantity to be dispensed, etc.).

B. What action should you take when a patient requests a refill of a prescription that does not have refills authorized?

C. What factors should the technician consider when evaluating the authenticity of a prescription/ medication order?

D. What factors should the technician consider when evaluating the accuracy and completeness of a prescription/medication order?

E. Why is the time of day when a medication order is written important in the institutional setting? Discuss examples of problems that could occur when time is not included on the order.

F. What action should you take when the pharmacy receives a prescription faxed from a patient or a patient's representative?

VIII. Sample Questions

A. What information is required on prescription orders but is not required on medication orders?

1. Patient information

2. Date

3. Dosage form

4. Quantity to be dispensed

5. All of the above are required on medication orders.

B. Prescriptions and medication orders must contain which of the following:

   1. Generic name of the drug

   2. Trade name of the drug

   3. Manufacturer of the prescribed drug

   4. Either 1 or 2

   5. All of the above

C. True or false?

   1. Telephone orders for new prescriptions may be received only by a registered pharmacist or, in some states, by a supervised pharmacy intern, but technicians may telephone prescribers for the authorization of refills.

   2. If the prescriber writes "no refills" or "NR" on the prescription order, the prescription may never be refilled.

D. Which of the following products are commercially available?

   1. Alendronate 70 mg solution

   2. Clarithromycin 500 mg tablets

   3. Benazepril hydrochloride 30 mg tablets

   4. Fluconazole 400 mg injection

   5. Idarubicin 10 mg capsules

   6. Simvastatin 60 mg tablets

   7. Albuterol sulfate 2 mg/5 ml oral syrup

   8. Cyclobenzaprine 100 mg tablets

   9. Prednisone 50 mg tablets

   10. Indomethacin 50 mg suppositories

   11. Nortriptyline 20 mg capsules

   12. Clindamycin 300 mg tablets

13. Felodipine 10 mg tablets

14. Etodolac 300 mg tablets

15. Timolol maleate 0.25% solution

16. Digoxin 5 mg tablet

17. Phenobarbital 15 mg tablet

E. Transcribe the following abbreviated instructions into readable directions as they should appear on a prescription label. Include leading verbs (take, inject, etc.).

1. ii tab. p.o. q.i.d.

2. i cap. a.c. & h.s.

3. 5 mg IM q.3–4h p.r.n. nausea

4. i gtt. o.d. q.12h

5. ii–iii gtt. a.u. t.i.d.

6. i gtt. a.u. b.i.d.

F. Which of the following describes routes of drug administration?

1. Suppository

2. Solution

3. Intravenous

4. Answers 1 and 2

5. All of the above

G. What instruction might be included on the prescription label for a suspension?

1. Shake well

2. Keep refrigerated

3. Apply to affected areas three times daily

    4.   Answers 1 and 2

    5.   All of the above

Answers appear on page 143.

Notes:

Chapter Two

Patient Information/
Profile Systems

I. Key Terms and Concepts

A. Patient profile
   1. A record containing information pertaining to a specific patient including demographic information, medical history, medication use chronology, allergies, and chronic illnesses.

B. Diagnosis
   1. The identified disease or health condition determined by the prescriber through assessment of the patient's signs and symptoms.

C. Psychosocial factors
   1. Involving both psychological and social aspects; relating social conditions to mental health.

D. Socioeconomic factors
   1. Of, relating to, or involving a combination of social and economic factors.

E. Desired therapeutic outcome
   1. The desired health result of drug therapy. The outcome may be an end result (e.g., complete cure of the disease), a goal related to incurable but controllable disease states (e.g., lowering and maintaining blood pressure to an acceptable level in a hypertensive patient), or a general goal of therapy (e.g., an appropriate level of sedation prior to surgery).

II. Assisting the Pharmacist in Obtaining Patient Information to Be Entered in the Patient Profile

A. Obtaining patient information
   1. At the direction of the pharmacist, technicians may be required to ask patient/patient's representative, prescriber, or other health professional for information about the patient. This information is important to the patient's use of a specific drug or drug regimen and is used to create or update the patient profile. Technicians should possess good communication skills and be knowledgeable about appropriate patient interviewing techniques to obtain accurate information.

B. Patient profiles
1. Patient profiles may be manual or computerized records. The following information may be included in a patient profile:
   a. Patient information
      (1) Ambulatory/outpatient setting
         (a) Patient's name, birth date, address, telephone number, pertinent insurance reimbursement information

      (2) Institutional/inpatient setting
         (a) Patient's name, birth date, address, height, weight, identification number, room number, primary physician

2. Diagnosis

3. Desired therapeutic outcome

4. Medication use
   a. The patient's medication history and current medication use (including nonprescription drugs) is critical to assessing the appropriateness of therapy. This information may be used to detect potential drug interactions, possible allergies, medication duplication, and other potential problems. The outpatient profile should include a chronology of medication refills.

5. Allergies
   a. The patient's history of allergies may predict potential allergies to similar drugs.

6. Adverse reactions
   a. The patient's history of adverse reactions may help predict potential adverse reactions to similar drugs.

7. Medical history
   a. This includes a chronology of past and current medical conditions.

8. Psychosocial history
   a. This is important because of its potential influence on patient compliance, drug misuse, drug abuse, and other factors. In some cases, the pharmacist may need to give the patient additional instructions or counseling.

9. Patient characteristics/special considerations
   a. These include characteristics that require special attention when processing the patient's prescriptions. Addressing these factors will help prevent potential problems (e.g., compliance, drug misuse). Patients with limitations may require special labeling, packaging, auxiliary materials (e.g., instructions written in large print or in another language), or counseling by the pharmacist. Examples include:
      (1) Physical characteristics
         (a) Visual impairment

(b) Hearing impairment

(c) Other physical disability

(2) Sociological characteristics
(a) Foreign language

(b) Cultural or religious beliefs

10. Socioeconomic history

11. Reimbursement mechanisms and third-party-payer information
   a. This function includes questioning the patient/patient's representative about the payment method, and assessing the eligibility of the patient and the prescribed product for reimbursement from the patient's third-party payer.

C. Collecting data to monitor patient outcomes
   1. At the direction of the pharmacist, technicians may collect data that will help the pharmacist monitor patient outcomes. Tests may include:
      a. Blood pressure measurements in those with preexisting or suspected hypertension

      b. Glucose (blood sugar) levels in diabetics, those suspected of having diabetes, or pregnant women who have had problems with elevated glucose levels

      c. Blood lipid analysis (cholesterol, low-density lipoproteins [LDL], high-density lipoproteins [HDL], etc.)

III. Entering Patient Information in the Patient Profile

A. New patients
   1. Patient profiles are generated for every patient receiving medications from the pharmacy department. Working with the pharmacist, technicians may be asked to create a profile for each new patient who receives a prescription from the pharmacy.

B. Patients with existing profiles
   1. Updating the medical record/patient profile
      a. Because the patient's health status and/or response to medications may change, patient profiles must be updated as often as necessary. The patient/patient's representative may not automatically volunteer this information; therefore, at the direction of the pharmacist, technicians may interview patients about possible changes in their health condition or medication use. Any of the items listed in the patient profile may need to be updated. Changes in patient information other than demographics (e.g., address) should be brought to the pharmacist's attention immediately so that the patient may be counseled appropriately. The most common changes include:

(1) Patient information. Ask the patient/patient's representative whether this information is correct and current.

(2) Diagnosis or desired therapeutic outcome. Has anything changed regarding the patient's disease or condition? Are there any new problems?

(3) Medication use. Is the patient still using the medications listed in the patient profile? Have any new prescription or nonprescription medications been added to the regimen?

(4) Allergies. Has the patient experienced allergic symptoms that may be related to current drug therapy?

(5) Adverse reactions. Has the patient experienced adverse reactions that may be related to current drug therapy?

(6) Reimbursement mechanisms and third-party-payer information. Is this information correct and current?

(7) Medication duplication. When updating the patient profile, it is important to be aware of the possibility of medication duplication. If discovered, the pharmacist should be notified immediately.

(8) Drug interactions. Be aware of the potential for drug interactions. Prescription drugs may interact with other prescription drugs, nonprescription drugs, food, and some laboratory tests.

IV. Chapter Summary

A. Developing and maintaining patient profile systems is a primary responsibility of technicians in both inpatient and outpatient settings.

B. Technicians must be knowledgeable about the patient information that is included in profiles and important changes that require special attention by the pharmacist.

C. Pharmacy technicians may assist the pharmacist in obtaining patient information by conducting interviews with patients or their representatives, and with health care professionals. To do this effectively, technicians must possess good communication skills and be proficient in various interviewing techniques. Obtaining information about a patient's diagnosis, desired therapeutic outcome, medication use, allergies, and other pertinent data is essential to the provision of complete pharmaceutical care.

D. Performing tests for elevated blood pressure, glucose, and cholesterol helps the pharmacist monitor the patient's therapeutic outcome. The technician can play a key role in this type of monitoring.

V. Questions for Discussion

A. Accepting new prescriptions/medication orders may require the technician to interview the patient/patient's representative about certain types of information.

    1. What types of questions should be asked of a new patient?

    2. What questions should be asked of a patient who has an existing patient profile?

B. Describe examples of psychosocial factors that may be important to consider when obtaining patient information for the patient profile.

C. How do a patient's psychosocial history and socioeconomic status affect the patient's ability to adhere to a prescribed therapeutic regimen?

D. Discuss ways the pharmacy technician can increase compliance in patients with physical disabilities.

E. Describe examples of medication and/or medication class duplication.

F. Discuss the importance of good communication skills in patient interviewing. What communication skills are most important?

G. Describe symptoms associated with an allergic reaction.

VI. Sample Questions

A. True or false?

    1. Nonprescription drugs should not be included in the patient profile.

    2. Patient profiles are created for every patient for whom a prescription/medication order is presented to the pharmacy.

    3. Changes in patient information other than demographics should be brought to the attention of the supervising pharmacist.

    4. Obtaining patient information to enter in the patient profile is almost never performed by the pharmacy technician.

B. When updating the patient profile, the technician may ask about all of the following types of information except:

   1. Patient's use of nonprescription medications

   2. Changes in insurance coverage

   3. Other prescriptions that the patient is receiving that are being provided by the physician or other pharmacies

   4. Laboratory tests the patient is scheduled to undergo

   5. All of the above types of information are important to be included in the patient profile

Answers appear on page 143.

Notes:

Chapter Three

Processing Prescriptions and Medication Orders

I. Key Terms and Concepts

A. Pharmacology
   1. The science that deals with the origin, nature, chemistry, effects, and uses of drugs

B. Compounding
   1. The act or process of combining two or more drug products or chemicals into a single preparation

C. Controlled substances
   1. Drugs that are regulated under the Controlled Substances Act, a federal law enacted in 1970. It regulates the prescribing and dispensing of drugs of abuse, according to five schedules (designated I, II, III, IV, and V) on the basis of their abuse potential, medical acceptance, and ability to produce dependence (addiction). The law also established a regulatory system for the manufacture, storage, and transport of the drugs in each schedule. Drugs covered by this act include opium and its derivatives, opiates, hallucinogens, depressants, stimulants, and anabolic steroids.

D. Sterile
   1. Aseptic; free from microorganisms and not producing microorganisms; containing no bacterial or viral contaminants

E. Intravenous admixtures
   1. Intravenous solutions compounded with two or more ingredients (i.e., one or more additives mixed with the primary intravenous solution)

F. Laminar airflow hood
   1. Equipment used for the preparation of sterile products that provides filtered air, flowing horizontally or vertically, to prevent contamination by microorganisms. Horizontal airflow hoods are generally used in the preparation of most products. Vertical airflow hoods are used for the preparation of cytotoxic drugs to protect the operator from exposure to these agents.

G. Cytotoxic agents/cytotoxins
   1. An agent that has a specific toxic action upon cells of susceptible organs. Cytotoxic agents are commonly used to treat many forms of cancer (neoplasms).

H. Antineoplastic agents
   1. An agent that is used to treat neoplasms (cancers)

I. Enteral nutrition products
   1. Nutritional formulations that substitute for food in patients who are unable to eat. Patients receive nutrition through a feeding tube that enters the gastrointestinal tract through the esophageal route or a surgically implanted port.

II. Understanding Drug Actions and Uses

A. Pharmacology and drug classifications
   1. Technicians should be knowledgeable about drug actions and pharmacological classifications.

III. Entering Prescription or Medication Order Information in the Patient Profile

A. Entering new prescription/medication information in an existing patient profile or creating a new patient profile is usually the first step in processing prescriptions/medication orders. Strict attention to detail when performing this function is critical because entry errors can directly affect patient safety. This function may also provide input into other systems. For example, entering the prescription/medication order into a computerized patient profile may simultaneously generate a prescription label, update the drug inventory record, create an entry into a "want book" or other ordering system, and update or change information in other databases. Steps to follow when entering new prescription/medication information include:

   1. Verify the patient's name and/or identification number. If the patient already has an existing profile, confirm that the patient information on the new order matches the patient information on the profile. If no patient profile is found, a new profile must be created. For a complete discussion about information included in patient profiles, see Chapter Two.

   2. Compare the new order with the patient profile. Look for medication duplication (the patient is already receiving the drug), drug class duplication, or other possible problems. If problems are discovered, the pharmacist should be notified immediately before proceeding.

   3. Enter the date, drug name, dosage form, quantity to be dispensed, directions for use, and number of refills, if any.

   4. Enter the prescriber information and the initials of the technician and supervising pharmacist dispensing the medication (how this information is entered may vary, depending on the pharmacy).

   5. Enter the reimbursement mechanism or third-party-payer information.

   6. Enter other information as required by the pharmacy's policies and procedures.

IV. Selecting Appropriate Product(s) to Be Dispensed

A. Selecting the appropriate drug to be dispensed for a prescription or medication order
   1. Prescriptions and medication orders should be filled from the original order to minimize errors. While filling the order, the technician must meticulously scrutinize the information that has been entered in the patient profile and on the prescription label, carefully comparing it with the original prescription/medication order.

B. Selecting the manufacturing source of the product(s) to be dispensed for a prescription or medication order. Prescriptions and medication orders may be written in two ways:

   1. Generic terminology
      a. When a pharmaceutical manufacturer's patent expires for a proprietary drug, other companies may obtain approval from the Food and Drug Administration (FDA) to manufacture and market their own version of the drug. Because of individual policies and purchasing contracts, each pharmacy may have a preferred manufacturing source for different generic drugs. When a prescription or medication order is written in generic terminology, the selection of which product to dispense usually depends on which manufacturer is the preferred source for that particular drug. The preferred source may also differ depending on the drug (e.g., the preferred source for hydrochlorothiazide tablets may be the ABC Company's generic brand, while the XYZ Company's generic acetaminophen may be the preferred generic product).

   2. Trade- or brand-name terminology
      a. Appropriate methods for processing prescriptions and medication orders written in trade-name terminology depend on policies and procedures related to several factors including state laws, third-party payers, and individual pharmacies or institutions.

         (1) Institutions. The pharmacy and therapeutics committee is usually charged with developing policies related to the use of drug products within the institution and creating formularies on the basis of these decisions. The formulary restricts which drugs a physician may prescribe and gives the pharmacy department authority to substitute a generic equivalent for a trade-name product if one is available. Therefore, when a medication order is written in trade-name terminology, it is common practice for the order to be filled with the preferred generic equivalent. If no generic equivalent exists (and the drug is on the formulary), the order is filled with the trade-name product.

         (2) Community and ambulatory pharmacies. Each pharmacy may have its own set of policies and procedures, in addition to preferred generics as mentioned above. Most commonly, third-party payers dictate whether the prescription will be filled (some medications are not covered) and how they will be filled (trade name or generic). Most payers require generic substitution when available. If a generic equivalent is available, it is common practice for the technician or pharmacist to ask the patient or the patient's representative if he or she will accept a generic substitute. If the patient or patient's representative prefers the trade-name version that is not approved by his or her particular health insurance company, the patient will usually have to pay the difference in price to the pharmacy.

C. Obtaining medications or devices from inventory. After determining the manufacturing source of the product(s) to be dispensed, obtain the medications or devices from inventory.

D. Calibrating equipment needed to prepare or compound the prescription or medication order. As an important quality control measure, equipment used for measuring or compounding prescriptions and medication orders should be calibrated regularly to ensure accuracy. Each pharmacy department has policies and procedures that describe calibration methods and schedules to follow to ensure that equipment is maintained on a routine basis.

V. Preparing and Dispensing Medications to Fill Prescriptions and Medication Orders

A. Dispensing finished dosage forms
   1. This includes measuring or counting finished dosage forms according to instructions on the original prescription or medication order.

B. Calculations
   1. At the direction of the pharmacist, the technician may assist in performing and/or verifying pharmaceutical calculations. A thorough discussion of calculations is presented in Section V.

C. Preparing intravenous admixtures and other sterile products
   1. Procedures for the preparation of intravenous admixtures and other sterile products can be found in a variety of sources. See Section V for calculations related to the preparation of intravenous solutions.

D. Compounding medications for dispensing according to prescription formula or instructions
   1. At the direction of the pharmacist, technicians may be asked to assist in the compounding function. See Section V for a discussion of calculations related to compounding preparations.

E. Recording preparation of medication in various dosage forms
   1. Information describing how the prescription was prepared should be documented on the prescription or medication order and on the patient profile.

F. Recording preparation of controlled substances for dispensing
   1. By law, controlled substances require a strict inventory control system, and comprehensive documentation is required to record the dispensing of controlled substances as both established dosage forms and as ingredients of compounded preparations. Inventory control records are usually organized according to drug name and dosage form (i.e., each product has its own record). The following information may be required for adequate documentation:
      a. Date the drug was removed from inventory

      b. Amount of drug that was removed from inventory

      c. How the drug was used (e.g., in the preparation of a cough syrup)

    d. Patient and auxiliary information
      (1) Ambulatory/outpatient setting
        (a) Patient name, prescription number, prescriber

      (2) Institutional/inpatient setting
        (a) Patient name, room number, identification number

      (3) Technician and pharmacist initials

      (4) Other information

VI. Preparing Intravenous Admixtures and Other Sterile Products

Technicians may help institutionalized patients, and sometimes outpatients, by preparing sterile intravenous fluids containing drugs, vitamins, or other nutrients.

A. Sterile/aseptic technique
Compounding intravenous solutions, other types of injections (intramuscular, subcutaneous, etc.), ophthalmic and otic products, and other preparations that will be instilled directly into the patient's body tissues (e.g., irrigation solutions) requires strict adherence to aseptic technique to prevent contamination by microorganisms.

1. Each institution and ambulatory pharmacy has written policies describing the proper use of aseptic technique. This type of compounding is usually done in a separate sterile compounding room or in a specially designated area in the pharmacy. Correct use of this technique involves proper attire, efficient hand washing, sterilization of the surface (horizontal or vertical laminar airflow hood), aseptic preparation of the sterile products, and maintaining the sterility of the compounding area.
    a. Proper attire for sterile technique
      (1) Proper attire for pharmacists and technicians preparing sterile products consists of a sterile gown, sterile gloves, a face mask to cover the nose and mouth, and a cap to contain and cover the hair.

    b. Hand washing
      (1) The first step technicians must take before preparing sterile products is hand washing. Hands must be cleaned thoroughly using chlorhexidine or another disinfectant.

    c. Sterilization of the compounding surface
      (1) The sterilizing agent may vary with each institution or pharmacy. Ethyl alcohol (ethanol) and isopropyl alcohol (isopropanol or "rubbing alcohol") are the most commonly used agents. Alcohol is poured in a thick layer on the hood surface, wiped down with sterile gauze from back to front, and left wet until it evaporates. Leaving the compounding surface wet allows enough time for the alcohol to kill microorganisms that may be on the surface.

      d. Sterilization of the injection sites on the additive containers
          (1) Similarly, the injection site on the additive vial is saturated with an alcohol preparation. The site is then wiped with sterile gauze to clean the area where the needle is inserted to inject, reconstitute, and withdraw the additive.

      e. Maintaining the sterility of materials used to prepare aseptic product
          (1) While preparing aseptic products, care must be taken to keep all surfaces and materials sterile, and to ensure that they do not come into contact with other surfaces that may not be sterile, or may be contaminated with other medications or substances.

      f. Maintaining the sterility of the compounding area
          (1) The sterile compounding room or area must be scrupulously and continually maintained to ensure that all products are prepared in a completely aseptic environment. Mandatory periodic tests are conducted to ensure that this area is maintained properly and is contamination-free.

  B. Compounding sterile preparations
    1. Additives
      a. Many drugs are stored in the pharmacy as sterile powders that must be reconstituted. With the use of aseptic technique, an appropriate amount of diluent (most commonly normal saline) is injected into the vial, the container is shaken, and then left on the hood surface until every particle of the powder is dissolved and the resultant solution is clear. It is then withdrawn from the vial and injected into a larger volume sterile solution. In some instances, the medication is withdrawn and dispensed in a labeled syringe to be injected directly into the patient, or into another IV the patient is receiving. Drugs that are available as solutions do not require reconstitution and may be withdrawn and added to the larger volume solution immediately.

    2. Preventing cross-contamination
      a. While aseptic technique prevents bacterial contamination, it also guards against cross-contamination between two or more drugs. This is important to prevent serious and potentially fatal allergic reactions. With the use of aseptic technique, the syringe used to dilute or withdraw one medication is never used to dilute or withdraw another drug. Similarly, materials used in the compounding of one drug must not touch containers or other materials used to prepare a different medication.

    3. Antineoplastic chemotherapy agents
      a. Most sterile products are prepared in a *horizontal* laminar airflow hood that directs filtered air horizontally toward the operator or technician to protect against contamination by microorganisms. Some chemotherapeutic agents used to treat cancer (neoplasms) are cytotoxic and can be hazardous to the operator. For this reason, these agents are prepared in a *vertical* laminar airflow hood, which directs filtered air vertically (from top to bottom of the hood) to protect the operator from possible adverse effects that may occur from exposure to these agents. Chapter 5 provides detailed information about the handling of chemotherapeutic agents.

4. Enteral products
   a. Most enteral products are manufactured and ready for use. The technician may be responsible for calculations and sterile compounding when a specific formulation is requested that is not commercially available.

VII. Packaging Preparations

A. Prescriptions
   1. Prescription preparations are usually packaged according to the requirements of the specific drug and/or dosage form. Most preparations, regardless of dosage form, are packaged and dispensed in containers that protect the drug from light, which can hasten the degradation of drug products.

B. Medication orders
   1. Unit-dose packaging
      a. Unit-dose packaging is employed for most drugs dispensed in the institutional setting. When not commercially available, the pharmacy department may use special equipment to package "bulk" medications into unit-dose forms.

   2. Multiple-dose packaging
      a. Drugs may be dispensed in "bulk" (more than a single dosage, sometimes several days' supply of medication). Multiple-dose packaging is most commonly used for drugs not commercially available in unit-dose packaging and not used by the hospital in sufficient quantity to make repackaging into unit-dose forms feasible. These products will require labeling consistent with the requirements of prescription labels.
         (1) Single-day (24-hour) supply. The pharmacy department may dispense a 24-hour supply of the drug in a labeled prescription vial. This is most commonly used for oral dosage forms.

         (2) Multiple-day supply. For some dosage forms, it is not reasonable to attempt repackaging into a single-day supply (e.g., creams, ointments not available in unit-dose packages).

   3. Packaging of sterile products
      a. Sterile products intended for intravenous or intramuscular injection are usually prepared by adding medications or nutrients to a sterile solution in the final container that will be aseptically sealed and dispensed. Sometimes, transferring solutions through intravenous tubing to the final container is required. A few preparations must be filtered before dispensing. The technician should be proficient in these techniques and knowledgeable about the individual processes required for each medication.

VIII. Labeling Prescriptions and Medication Orders

A. Prescriptions. Prescriptions should be labeled with the following information:
   1. Name and address of pharmacy

   2. Date the prescription was filled

   3. Prescription number

   4. Drug name (generic or trade), strength, and quantity

   5. Directions for patient (administration route, schedule, duration)

   6. Patient's name

   7. Prescriber's name

   8. Expiration date

   9. Number of refills (if authorized)

   10. Lot number

   11. Pharmacist's initials

   12. Auxiliary labels providing additional information on storage, administration guidelines, cautions, etc.

   13. Other information required by state or federal laws
       a. Controlled substances
          (1) Federal transfer label

B. Medication orders
   1. Unit-dose medications should be labeled with the following information (commercially available unit-dose products are already labeled by the manufacturer with the appropriate information, although auxiliary labels may be needed for some drugs):
       a. Drug name and strength

       b. Lot number

       c. Expiration date

       d. Directions for administration if necessary (e.g., for intramuscular injection only)

       e. Auxiliary labels if necessary (storage, administration guidelines, cautions, etc.)

2. Multiple-dose packages should be labeled with the following information:
    a. Patient's name and room number

    b. Drug name, strength, and quantity

    c. Directions for administration

    d. Lot number

    e. Expiration date

    f. Auxiliary labels if necessary (storage, administration guidelines, cautions, etc.)

3. Sterile products should be labeled with the same information required on multiple-dose packages (see 2, above).

IX. Verifying Dispensing and Labeling Accuracy

A. Performing intermediate checks during processing of the prescription/medication order
    1. Performing intermediate checks is critical during the dispensing and labeling process. Technicians must pay careful attention to the specific details of the prescription/medication order, continually comparing the original order, label, patient profile, and the drug selected for accuracy.

    2. The technician may also be called upon to verify the measurements, preparation, and/or packaging of medications produced by other technicians.

B. Pharmacist authorization
    1. Authorization from the supervising pharmacist must be obtained and documented before prescriptions or medication orders are dispensed.

C. Technician authorization
    1. The final check/verification of the prescription or medication order may be performed by a supervising technician if allowed by law.

X. Compiling Patient Information Materials

A. At the direction of the pharmacist, the technician may be responsible for collecting supplemental patient information materials (e.g., patient package inserts, computer-generated information, videos) to be dispensed with the prescription/medication order.

XI. Delivering Medications to the Patient or the Patient's Representative

A. The technician should be familiar with the following functions related to the delivery of medications to patients. Specific policies and procedures governing these functions may vary, depending on the institution or pharmacy.

    1. Storing medications prior to distribution

        a. The technician should be familiar with the pharmacy's policies regarding storage of medications prior to distribution and also be knowledgeable about which medications require special storage conditions (e.g., refrigeration).

    2. Delivering medication to the patient or patient's representative

        a. Ambulatory/outpatient setting

            (1) In most states, technicians are authorized to make the offer for pharmacist consultation.

        b. Institutional/inpatient setting

            (1) Place medication in the unit-dose cart.

            (2) Deliver medication to the patient-care unit.

        c. Pharmacy benefits management company or mail-order setting

            (1) Package and ship pharmaceuticals, durable and nondurable medical equipment, devices, and supplies (including hazardous substances and investigational products) to patient/patient's representative.

    3. Recording distribution of prescription medications

    4. Recording distribution of controlled substances

XII. Determining Charges and Obtaining Compensation for Services

A. Calculating charges

    1. Charges for prescriptions and medication orders vary depending on a specific pharmacy department's policies and third-party reimbursement plans. A review of calculations related to pricing prescriptions is presented in Chapter Fourteen.

B. Communicating with third-party payers to determine or verify coverage

    1. The technician may be responsible for contacting third-party payers to verify the patient's eligibility for coverage.

    2. The technician may be responsible for contacting third-party payers for prior approval of nonformulary drugs and supplies.

C. Obtaining compensation

    1. Ambulatory/outpatient setting

        a. Payment from the patient or patient's representative

            (1) In the ambulatory setting, the first step in obtaining compensation is through receipt of a payment or partial payment (copayment) from the patient or the patient's representative.

   b. Reimbursement from third-party payers
      (1) For patients covered by third-party plans, the second step in obtaining compensation is through contact with the specific company providing prescription benefit coverage for the patient. The technician may be responsible for completing the appropriate paperwork (or computer-generated forms) to request reimbursement from various third-party payers.

      (2) Identify and resolve problems with rejected claims (e.g., incorrect days' supply, incorrect patient identification number).

      (3) Communicate with third-party payers and patient or the patient's representative to rectify rejected third-party claims.

2. Institutional/inpatient setting
   a. Patient billing
      (1) The pharmacy technician may be responsible for billing drug charges to the patient's account. The actual task of direct billing to patients and third-party payers is usually done by the institution's accounting department.

XIII. Providing Supplemental Information, as Indicated

A. The technician should ask all patients if counseling by a pharmacist is desired.

B. At the direction of the pharmacist, the technician may be responsible for giving the patient supplemental information materials along with the prescription/medication order.
   1. Patient package inserts (PPIs) are usually given to all patients, but FDA regulations require that PPIs must be provided to patients receiving the following medications:
      a. Oral contraceptives

      b. Products containing estrogenic drugs

      c. Products containing progestational drugs

      d. Isotretinoin

      e. Intrauterine devices

      f. Isoproterenol inhalation products

   2. Videos

XIV. Chapter Summary

    A. Processing prescriptions and medication orders is a multifaceted operation requiring knowledge of many different aspects of pharmacy technician practice.

    B. Preparation of sterile products and admixtures requires the technician to be proficient in the use of aseptic technique and knowledgeable about process requirements specific to each medication.

    C. Strict attention to detail must be followed while performing multiple tasks, including reviewing the patient profile; selecting, preparing, packaging, and labeling the appropriate product to fill the order; verifying dispensing and labeling accuracy through intermediate checks; calculating patient charges and obtaining compensation from third-party payers; and delivering the product and supplemental patient information to the patient or patient's representative.

XV. Questions for Discussion

    A. Before the unit-dose system was developed, institutions typically dispensed a 5-day supply of each regular medication, packaged and labeled in a prescription vial. Discuss the advantages and disadvantages of each system.

    B. What factors should be considered when selecting the appropriate product to be dispensed for a prescription/medication order?

    C. Describe various types of packaging and discuss the advantages and disadvantages of each.

    D. Describe the use of aseptic technique and processes used to prepare sterile products.

XVI. Sample Questions

    A. True or false?

        1. In the outpatient setting, pharmacists must authorize all prescription orders before the medications are dispensed to the patient; however, in the institutional setting, pharmacist authorization is not required if the technician gives the drug directly to a registered nurse because nurses have the same authority.

        2. In the institutional setting, multiple-dose packaging is preferred for most oral dosage forms.

        3. A supervising pharmacist must continually observe a technician preparing sterile products.

B. Unit-dose medications should be labeled with all of the following information except:

1. Lot number

2. Prescriber's name

3. Expiration date

4. Name of medication

5. Strength of medication

C. All of the following medications require patient package inserts to be dispensed with the prescription except:

1. Premarin®

2. Brevicon®

3. Ogen®

4. Accutane®

5. Vagitrol®

D. When selecting the appropriate product to fill a prescription/medication order, confusion caused by similar drug names can result in dispensing errors. Match each generic name with the appropriate brand name:

1. Escitalopram	a.	Flexeril®
2. Glimeprimide	b.	Allegra®
3. Allopurinol	c.	Lexapro®
4. Chlorpromazine	d.	Narcan®
5. Atorvastatin	e.	Amaryl®
6. Fexofenadine	f.	Compazine®
7. Cyclobenzaprine	g.	Diovan®
8. Methyldopa	h.	Proscar®
9. Valsarten	i.	Lipitor®
10. Naloxone	j.	Aldomet®
11. Prochlorperazine	k.	Thorazine®
12. Finasteride	l.	Zyloprim®

    E. Aseptic technique:

        1. Is used exclusively for the compounding of injectable preparations

        2. Prevents cross-contamination between two or more drugs

        3. May include the injection of ethyl alcohol into powdered additives to sterilize the preparations

        4. May prevent some allergic reactions in patients receiving injectable drugs

        5. Answers 2 and 4 are correct

Answers appear on page 143.

Notes:

Section II

Maintaining Medication and Inventory Control Systems

Includes activities related to medication and supply purchasing, inventory control, and preparation and distribution of medications according to approved policies and procedures

Chapter Four

Medication Distribution and Inventory Control Systems

I.   Key Terms and Concepts

A. Inventory
1. Pharmacy products or merchandise (drugs, devices, etc.) that is available to meet future demand

B. Inventory control
1. A procedure whereby products are purchased in sufficient quantity to meet the anticipated demands of purchasers while controlling inventory size to generate optimal profits

C. Turnover rate
1. The number of times a product is purchased, sold, and replaced during a specific accounting period. Inventory turnover is also discussed in Chapter Fourteen.

II. Ordering Pharmaceuticals, Durable Medical Equipment, Devices, and Supplies

A. Identifying products to be ordered
1. Determining which products to order depends on the inventory-purchasing procedures of each individual pharmacy. Factors that influence ordering decisions include expected inventory turnover rate, manufacturing sources of products, and the purchase price of a particular product.

B. Entering information on products to be ordered
1. Pharmaceuticals
   a. Drug name and manufacturer
      (1) Generic name/manufacturer name

      (2) Trade name if applicable

   b. Strength and dosage form of medication (tablets, capsules, solutions, suspensions, injections, suppositories, etc.)

   c. Type of packaging (unit dose or bulk packaging)

      d. Quantity contained in unit desired (e.g., 100's, 16 oz.)

      e. Number of units

  2. Equipment, devices, and supplies
      a. Name and manufacturer of product

      b. Strength or size (if applicable) of product

      c. Quantity contained in unit desired

      d. Number of units

      e. Other information as required

C. Identifying appropriate sources. Appropriate sources for various products are determined by each pharmacy's ordering policies.
  1. Wholesale drug distributors

  2. Manufacturers

  3. Other pharmacies

D. Expediting emergency orders
  1. The technician should be knowledgeable about the timetables for delivery of goods ordered from various sources so that drugs needed quickly can be obtained from the most desirable source in accordance with pharmacy policies and procedures.

  2. In an emergency, the usual preferred sources may not be feasible, and the pharmacy may need to borrow the product from a nearby pharmacy or institution.

III. Receiving Goods

A. Verifying specifications on original purchase orders

  1. Verifying products ordered versus products received. To ensure that the correct product was sent by the manufacturer or wholesale distributor, the technician must carefully scrutinize the order and confirm that the information is consistent in all the components: (a) the original purchase order or "want book," (b) the invoice received with the order, and (c) the products received in the order. The following information should be compared and verified in each of the components for appropriateness and accuracy:
      a. Drug name and manufacturer
          (1) Generic name/trade name

      b. Strength and dosage form of medication

    c. Appropriateness of packaging type (e.g., unit-dose versus bulk packaging)

    d. Quantity contained in unit desired (e.g., 100's, 16 oz.)

    e. Number of units received versus number ordered

  2. Documenting receipt of goods
    a. Pharmaceuticals, durable medical equipment, devices, and supplies
      (1) Notations on the invoice indicating receipt of appropriate products, or shortages, are usually written by the technician.

    b. Controlled substances
      (1) Receipt of controlled substances must be documented by the supervising pharmacist.

IV. Placing Pharmaceuticals, Durable Medical Equipment, Devices, and Supplies in Inventory

A. Products should be placed in inventory under proper storage conditions. The technician should be knowledgeable about which products require special storage conditions (e.g., refrigeration).

B. Products should be placed in inventory according to stock rotation procedures, with items that will expire soonest placed in front of items with later expiration dates.

V. Removing Pharmaceuticals, Durable Medical Equipment, Devices, and Supplies from Inventory

A. Identifying products to be removed from inventory
  1. Expired and discontinued products

  2. Slow-moving products

  3. Recalled products

VI. Repackaging Medications in Anticipation of Prescriptions and Medication Orders

A. Prepackaging finished dosage forms for dispensing (e.g., unit dose)
  1. Most drugs may be obtained in unit-dose packaging, but technicians may be responsible for repackaging some products. The technician should be familiar with the pharmacy's policies and procedures for repackaging to prevent shortages.

VII. Compounding Medications in Anticipation of Prescriptions and Medication Orders

A. Bulk compounding
1. Compounds not commercially available may be prescribed and dispensed on a regular basis. As a means of avoiding the time-consuming activity of compounding the medication for each order, a large quantity may be prepared in advance in anticipation of future prescription or medication orders. The technician should be familiar with the pharmacy's policies and procedures for bulk compounding to prevent shortages.

VIII. Maintaining Record-Keeping Systems for Changes Affecting Inventory Levels of Pharmaceuticals, Durable Medical Equipment, Devices, and Supplies

A. Recalls and returns
1. Documenting recalls and returns may require entering the following information into the inventory records:
   a. Date the product was removed from inventory

   b. Information to identify the product
      (1) Pharmaceuticals
         (a) Drug name, strength, dosage form, and quantity removed

      (2) Equipment, devices, and supplies
         (a) Product name, size, and any other pertinent information for identification

   c. Manufacturer of the product

   d. Lot number or identification number

   e. Purpose for removing the drug from inventory (e.g., manufacturer recall)

   f. Initials of technician and supervising pharmacist

   g. Other information as required by pharmacy policies

B. Repackaging and bulk compounding of pharmaceuticals
1. Documenting repackaging and bulk compounding may require entering the following information into the inventory records:
   a. Date the drug was removed from bulk inventory into the repackaged form or compounded product

   b. Drug name, strength, dosage form, and quantity used

   c. Lot number

    d. Initials of technician and supervising pharmacist

    e. Other information as required by pharmacy policies

IX. Maintaining Records of Controlled Substances

A. Recording controlled substances received and stored
    1. Documentation of this function may require the following information:
        a. Date the drug was received

        b. Drug name, strength, dosage form, and quantity received

        c. Initials of technician and supervising pharmacist

        d. Other information as required by pharmacy policies

B. Recording controlled substances removed from inventory
    1. Documentation of this function may require the following information:
        a. Date the drug was removed from inventory

        b. Drug name, strength, dosage form, and quantity removed

        c. Lot number

        d. Purpose for removing the drug from inventory (e.g., manufacturer recall)

        e. Initials of technician and supervising pharmacist

        f. Other information as required by pharmacy policies

X. Maintaining Policies and Procedures to Deter Theft and/or Drug Diversion

A. *Drug theft* and *drug diversion* are synonymous terms for illegally obtaining any medication; however, the drugs usually affected are controlled substances. The term *drug diversion* is generally used to describe health professionals stealing narcotics for personal use.

B. Drugs are stolen for many reasons, but three reasons predominate:
    1. Personal abuse or addiction

    2. Another person's abuse or addiction

    3. Resale

C. Pharmacy policies to deter theft often include the following:
  1. Storing controlled substances in a locked cabinet

  2. Conducting a physical inventory of controlled substances periodically and monitoring the inventory on an ongoing basis

  3. Maintaining records on controlled substances (see IX, above)

  4. Allowing only a licensed pharmacist into the pharmacy after hours for dispensing of medications

XI. Communicating Changes in Product Availability to Pharmacy Staff, Patients/Patients' Representatives, Physicians, and Other Health Care Professionals

A. Reasons for changes in product availability
  1. Recalls

  2. Formulary changes

  3. Discontinued products

  4. Manufacturer shortages

B. Methods for communicating product changes
  1. Personal communication
     a. Communicating with the patient or patient's representative

     b. Staff meetings

  2. Written communication
     a. Memorandum to staff and other health care professionals

     b. Pharmacy newsletter

     c. Institutional newsletter

XII. Collecting and Analyzing Data on the Quality of Pharmacy Products and Services

A. Routine monitoring of the pharmacy department's activities is necessary to ensure the quality of pharmacy products and services, and serves to identify existing and potential problems. Quality assurance activities include the collection and analysis of data on product preparation and distribution processes including:

1. Sterile product testing
   a. Evaluating processes used in the preparation and sterilization of products to ensure that sterile products are free from microbial contamination, particulate matter, and pyrogens. Various tests are used in this assessment.

2. Packaging unit-dose medications

3. Bulk compounding

4. Drug distribution activities
   a. Evaluating accuracy in filling and checking unit-dose medication carts

5. Record-keeping activities
   a. Evaluating or reviewing patient profiles, medication administration records, and other records related to the above processes

XIII. Chapter Summary

A. Monitoring medication distribution and inventory control systems is a primary responsibility of pharmacy technicians.

B. The technician should be knowledgeable about the pharmacy's policies and procedures related to ordering products, receiving goods, storing products in inventory, repackaging, bulk compounding, quality assurance activities, and record-keeping systems for all processes.

XIV. Questions for Discussion

A. What factors should be considered in determining which products should be ordered for the pharmacy?

B. What factors should be considered in determining what quantity of a particular product should be ordered?

C. What factors should be considered in identifying the appropriate supplier from which to order a particular product?

D. Discuss the differences between drug theft and drug diversion. What is the technician's role in deterring drug theft and diversion?

   E. Describe specific methods for collecting and analyzing data on the quality of pharmacy products and services.

XV. Sample Questions

   A. When medications are recalled by the manufacturer, all of the following steps should be followed except:
       1. Remove the recalled product from inventory.

       2. Destroy the remaining units of recalled product and document actions.

       3. Notify patients who are using the medication.

       4. Notify health care providers about the recall.

       5. All of the above steps should be followed.

   B. True or false?
       1. In institutional practice, all medications that are not available in unit-dose packaging must be repackaged.

       2. Schedule II controlled substances may not be repackaged into unit-dose form.

   C. Which of the following drugs should be stored in the refrigerator prior to dispensing?
       1. Reconstituted amoxicillin suspension

       2. Haloperidol solution

       3. Sulfamethoxazole/trimethoprim suspension

       4. Meperidine hydrochloride injection

       5. All of the above medications

   D. Match the drug with the condition under which it should be stored:
       a. Room temperature   b. Frozen   c. Refrigeration

       1. Aspirin suppositories

       2. Calcitonin-salmon nasal spray

       3. Acetaminophen suppositories

       4. Chlordiazepoxide injection

5. Diazepam injection

6. Lorazepam injection

7. L-Hyoscyamine sulfate drops

8. Succinyl choline powder

9. Neosporin genitourinary irrigant

10. Oral poliovirus vaccine

Answers appear on page 144.

Notes:

Section III

Processing and Handling of Specific Drug Categories

Includes activities related to protocols for processing and handling of specific drug categories, including:

- chemotherapeutic medications
- investigational drugs
- restricted drugs

Chapter Five

Processing and Handling Commercially Available Chemotherapeutic Medications
Processing Chemotherapeutic Medications
Available in Finished Dosage Forms

I. Key Terms and Concepts

A. Chemotherapy

Chemotherapy may refer to any type of drug therapy, but has been used particularly to describe drugs that kill a causative organism, usually, without harming the patient. Formerly used to describe antibacterial agents, the term *chemotherapy* has recently become associated with drugs used to treat cancer. Unlike radiopharmaceuticals and surgery, chemotherapeutic medications work systemically, traveling throughout the entire body instead of being confined to a particular area. This distribution enables the drug to reach cancer cells that may have spread to other parts of the body (metastasized). Topical chemotherapeutic drugs work at the site of application. Chemotherapeutic agents vary widely in chemical compostion, mechanism of action, modes of administration, and side effects.

B. Antineoplastic therapy

A general term for anticancer therapy, derived from the word *neoplasm*, defined as the growth of abnormal tissue (cancer).

1. Cytotoxic therapy

   a. Cytotoxic (cell-killing) agents are used to kill or arrest the growth of abnormal cancer cells. Most interfere with the cell's ability to grow or multiply.

   b. Commonly used chemotherapeutic agents
   More than 50 chemotherapy drugs are currently available. Some of the most commonly used agents are listed below:

Capecitabine (Xeloda®)	Chlorambucil (Leukeran®)
Cisplatin (Platinol®)	Cyclophosphamide (Cytoxan®)
Daunorubicin (Cerubidine®)	Doxorubicin (Adriamycin®)
Etoposide (VePesid®)	Fluorouracil (5-FU, Efudex®)
Meclorethamine (Mustargen®)	Melphalan (Alkeran®)
Mercaptopurine (Purinethol®)	Methotrexate (Trexall®)

   c. Adverse reactions

      (1) Cytotoxic drugs may not distinguish between a normal healthy cell and a cell that is cancerous; therefore, they may kill surrounding cells of healthy tissue.

(2) Cytotoxic agents target specific parts of the cell growth cycle, usually rapidly dividing cells that are common in cancer tumors. Unfortunately, normal healthy cells share some of these pathways and may be injured or killed by chemotherapy.

    (a) Some normal cell processes (blood cells, hair, and cells lining the gastrointestinal tract) are also rapidly dividing and may be damaged by chemotherapy. Many side effects are caused by adverse effects on these normal tissues.

(3) Cytotoxic drugs may be carcinogenic (causing cancer), teratogenic (causing birth defects), or mutagenic (causing genetic changes).

(4) The severity of adverse reactions depends on the individual drug. Nausea, vomiting, and hair loss are common with some drugs, whereas other more-serious side effects such as blood cell changes and organ damage may also occur.

(5) Newer drugs that target pathways used only by cancer cells are being developed, and some have already been approved by the Food and Drug Administration (FDA). These agents may be more effective and may cause fewer side effects.

2. Hormone therapy

Hormonal therapy adds, blocks, or removes hormones that stimulate the growth of cancer cells. Estrogen may promote the growth of breast cancer cells, so hormone therapy may be used to block the body's naturally occurring estrogen to stop the cancer cells from growing. Similarly, testosterone-blocking agents may slow or stop the growth of prostate cancer cells that depend on testosterone.

    a. Selective estrogen receptor modulators (SERMS)

        (1) Tamoxifen (Nolvadex®) molecules chemically resemble estrogen and bind to estrogen receptors, blocking estrogen from breast cancer cells. Unlike estrogen, tamoxifen does not stimulate breast cancer cell growth.

    b. Aromatase inhibitors block aromatase, an enzyme that is a major source of estrogen in many body tissues including breast, muscle, liver, and fat.

        (1) Anastrozole (Arimidex®)

        (2) Exemestane (Aromasin®)

        (3) Formestane (Lenatron®)

        (4) Letrozole (Femara®)

    c. Selective estrogen receptor downregulators (SERDs) block estrogen in all tissues in the body.

        (1) Fulvestrant (Faslodex®)

    d. Progestins usually are used as second- or third-line treatment of advanced breast cancer when tamoxifen fails.

        (1) Megestrol (Megace®)

e. Leuteinizing hormone-releasing hormone (LHRH) agonists prevent the testicles from producing testosterone and slow the growth of prostate cancer cells.
   (1) Goserelin (Zoladex®)

   (2) Leuprolide (Lupron®)

f. Antiandrogens block the effects of any remaining male hormones after orchiectomy or treatment with other testosterone-blocking agents that have eliminated testosterone production by the testicles. These drugs block male hormones produced by the adrenal gland.
   (1) Bicalutamide (Casodex®)

   (2) Flutamide (Eulexin®)

g. Estrogen stops the testicles from producing testosterone but is rarely used to treat prostate cancer because of its side effects.

h. Adverse reactions to hormone therapy
   Although fewer severe adverse effects occur with hormone therapy, side effects may occur, usually because of the decrease in levels of natural hormones. Hormonal agents generally do not require the special handling techniques required for cytotoxic chemotherapy agents.
   (1) Estrogen-blocking agents may cause hot flashes, bleeding and discharge, visual disturbances, increased risk for blood clots, and increased risk for uterine cancer with long-term therapy.

   (2) Testosterone-blocking agents may cause nausea, constipation or diarrhea, decreased appetite, dizziness, headache, insomnia, gynecomastia (swelling or tenderness of breasts), impotence, and decreased sex drive.

II. Processing and Handling of Chemotherapeutic Agents

A. Exceptions from handling of chemotherapeutic agents
   1. Pregnant or lactating women

   2. Male or female staff who are actively trying to conceive a child

   3. Personnel with a medical condition that may prohibit them from handling cytotoxic drugs

   4. Personnel who fail to meet competency requirements

B. Competency to handle and prepare cytotoxic drugs must be established.
   1. Training must be completed in accordance with the institution's guidelines/protocols.

   2. Personnel must demonstrate competency through written, oral, and/or practical testing.

III. Handling of Chemotherapeutic Drugs Commercially Available in Finished Dosage Forms

Although it is commonly believed that only injectable chemotherapeutic agents pose a risk to health care workers, the handling and dispensing of oral cytotoxic drugs are also a safety concern. Therefore, special precautions must be taken when handling and dispensing these agents.

A. Routes of exposure
    1. Inhalation of drug aerosols, droplets, or particles
        a. Aerosolization may occur by:
            (1) Crushing or splitting tablets

            (2) Opening capsules

            (3) Preparing liquids

            (4) Handling powders

        b. Absorption through skin or eye contact
            (1) Risks associated with handling oral dosage forms of cytotoxic drugs appear to be low, but potentially may increase with repeated exposure over several years.

        c. Ingestion through contact with contaminated food or food containers
            (1) Precautions for handling these agents include hygienic and decontamination procedures.

B. Protective apparel
    1. Gloves
        a. Gloves without powder are preferred because the powder may absorb the cytotoxic agent. Gloves should be changed regularly or after a tear, spill, or puncture. Technicians working in chemo-only areas should also change gloves hourly or sooner, as needed.

    2. Gowns, masks, eye protectors, and caps
        a. These may also be used, depending on the practice site and extent of exposure. Each facility will have specific practice and procedural guidelines.

C. Protective equipment
    1. Biological safety cabinet (BSC)
        a. An enclosed laminar hood for the preparation of cytotoxic drugs. The cabinet sustains a sterile vertical airflow and provides a shield to protect the operator from exposure to the agent.

        b. The BSC may be used for crushing, splitting, or packaging oral cytotoxic drugs.

D. Preparing and maintaining the work area
    1. The preparation or work area where chemotherapeutic drugs are stored or prepared must be a restricted area for authorized personnel only. Storing food, eating, and drinking in this area are prohibited.

    2. Apparel must not leave the preparation area and should be disposed of according to the practice site's hazardous waste disposal procedures.

IV. Receiving Chemotherapeutic Drugs

A. Manufacturers are required to label cytotoxic drugs, and most include padding to ensure safety if a container is broken.

    1. Gloves and other protective apparel (as needed) should be worn when receiving cytotoxic agents.

    2. Cytotoxic drugs should be separated from other drugs in the receiving area.

    3. Liquid spills should be handled according to the practice facility's policies and procedures.

V. Guidelines for Handling and Dispensing Cytotoxic Drugs

A. Technicians and other health care workers should wear gloves and other protective apparel when handling cytotoxic agents.

B. They should also use a designated counting tray and spatula to ensure cross-contamination of other drugs does not occur.

    1. Trays, spatulas, and immediate workspace should be wiped with a small amount of detergent, rinsed thoroughly, and then wiped with alcohol to ensure that drug residues are not left in the work area.

C. Waste from these agents should be disposed of in a puncture-proof cytotoxic waste container, including cotton from bottles, pads used to wipe surfaces, gloves, bottles, and vials. The disposal container should be clearly labeled as cytotoxic waste.

VI. Chapter Summary

A. Chemotherapeutic drugs are useful in the treatment of various cancers.

B. Most chemotherapeutic agents are cytotoxic, killing cancerous cells. Unfortunately, sometimes noncancerous cells are affected, resulting in adverse reactions beyond those expected.

C. The preparation and dispensing of chemotherapeutic agents may require special precautions, such as using protective apparel, protective equipment, and thorough decontamination procedures.

D. The technician should be familiar with guidelines for receiving, handling, and dispensing of these agents according to the practice site's written policies.

VII. Questions for Discussion

A. What is the most common mechanism of action of chemotherapeutic agents?

B. Why do chemotherapy drugs require special handling?

C. What types of protection should technicians use when handling cytotoxic agents?

D. Why are powder-free gloves preferred when handling cytotoxic drugs?

E. What specific mechanism of action is most responsible for side effects from cytotoxic drugs?

VIII. Sample Questions

A. What information must you know before handling any drug in the pharmacy?

1. Whether it has cytotoxic properties

2. Whether it has storage requirements

3. Whether special procedures or precautions are required for its handling and preparation

4. Whether special apparel should be worn while receiving and handling the drug

5. All of the above

B. Which of the following agents is not considered to be cytotoxic chemotherapy?

1. Fluorouracil (Efudex®)

2. Mercaptopurine (Purinethol®)

3. Methotrexate (Trexall®)

4. Tamoxifen (Nolvadex®))

5. They are all cytotoxic agents.

C. Knowledge of precautions for handling chemotherapeutic agents, and policies and procedures determined by a practice site is important because:

1. Long-term exposure may cause adverse effects in health care personnel.

2. The potential for cross-contamination is diminished.

3. Crushing or splitting tablets may increase exposure.

4. Special procedures must be followed if spills occur.

5. All of the above are correct.

D. True or false?

    1. All cytotoxic drugs kill cancerous cells only and have minimal effects on other areas.

    2. Exposure of health care personnel to cytotoxic agents over a long period of time is minimal if special precautions and procedures are followed.

    3. Unlike injectable agents, oral cytotoxic drugs do not pose a risk to health care personnel.

    4. Most practice sites have policies and procedures for handling cytotoxic agents.

    5. The entire inventory of cytotoxic drugs should always be stored in BSCs until ready for preparation and dispensing.

E. What *systemic* mechanism is mostly responsible for side effects from cytotoxic drugs?

    1. The drugs are irritating.

    2. Most chemotherapeutic agents cause drowsiness.

    3. Conventional chemotherapy targets rapidly dividing cells.

    4. Ataxia may occur when cytotoxic agents are prescribed in high doses.

    5. None of the above is correct.

F. What organ systems are most likely to be affected by conventional chemotherapy?

    1. White blood cells

    2. Gastrointestinal system

    3. Hair

    4. All of the above

    5. None of the above

Answers appear on page 144.

Notes:

Chapter Six

Collecting and Communicating Data on Investigational Drugs
Receiving and Processing Investigational Drugs

I. Key Terms and Concepts

A. Investigational drugs (ID)
   1. Drugs that have been studied in clinical trials but are not yet approved by the Food and Drug Administration (FDA) for use in the general population. FDA requires that studies in the larger community follow specific protocols, supervised by the principal investigator and monitors. Investigational drugs are prepared by pharmacists and technicians, following protocols for record keeping, storage, preparation, and dispensing. Investigational Drug Services (IDS), provided by pharmacy departments, are responsible for the oversight of all of these activities.

B. Principal investigator
   1. The principal investigator in a community or hospital setting is usually a physician specializing in the disease being studied.

C. Protocol
   1. A protocol is a plan that describes how an experiment or study should be conducted. Protocols also include guidelines for preparing and handling the investigational agent.

II. Investigational Drugs Overview

Investigational drug studies are conducted by physicians in various practice settings to gather information about the appropriate use, efficacy, dosage, and safety of drugs that are promising for treating particular diseases. These agents have already been tested in limited clinical trials and are now being tried in the larger community, usually in patients in whom other therapies have been unsuccessful or poorly tolerated because of side effects. The larger studies will provide more-extensive information about the efficacy and safety of these drugs.

The policies for procurement, storage, inventory control, destruction, and return of investigational drugs are usually consistent with policies for other prescription drugs. However, investigational agents require greater accountability and control procedures specified by federal agencies, sponsors of the study, and the Joint Commission on Accreditation of Healthcare Organizations. Protocols for each medication being studied accompany the product information provided to the pharmacy, and everyone in the pharmacy involved with the processing, compounding, or delivery of study drugs should be familiar with all of these protocols and procedures.

A. Processing and handling investigational dugs

    1. Procedures for handling and processing investigational drugs vary with each agent being investigated. Each drug is assigned specific instructions on preparation and handling, depending on its unique properties.

    2. Aspects to consider

       a. Stability

          (1) Because investigational drugs usually have not been thoroughly studied and widely manufactured, stability may be a major consideration in preparation, storage, and delivery. Some agents, especially intravenous solutions, degrade quickly and must be used in a few hours. Instructions describing appropriate preparation techniques, storage, and stability should be studied in advance.

       b. Toxicity

          (1) If the investigational drug is mutagenic or teratogenic, as with some chemotherapeutic agents, special handling is required and is described in the preparation instructions for chemotherapeutic agents. Also, see Chapter 5 for more information.

       c. Scheduling

          (1) Physicians participating in a community study need investigational drugs to be prepared and ready for administration to the patient, sometimes immediately or at different times on different days during the week. It is important to keep accurate records so that medications received by the physician or facility are prepared in time for appropriate administration and stored properly for future administration.

       d. Records

          (1) Record-keeping procedures for investigational drug programs follow guidelines set by federal agencies and investigators. In most instances, the physician or institution will provide the drug to the pharmacy for preparation. The pharmacy has the responsibility of documenting all information regarding receipt, storage conditions, handling procedures, and preparation techniques. Records also detail how and when the drug is delivered for administration, and ensure that schedules and protocols are followed. The pharmacy will record the following information about every investigational drug:

             (a) Date and time received. The log sheet is usually kept with the investigational drug stock to facilitate easy access and accountability. The National Institutes of Health Log Sheets are used for most drug studies. Sometimes, the study sponsor will require other forms, specific to a particular drug, to be used during the study.

             (b) Packing slip includes information on shipping, shipping contents (e.g., drug, diluents), principal investigator, and the protocol to be followed.

             (c) Proper storage, determined by temperature and lighting (refrigerated, nonrefrigerated, light sensitive), should be immediately noted. Investigational drugs should be kept in a permanent storage space, separate from other medications.

             (d) Investigational drugs will be labeled with drug name, strength, administration, expiration date, and the number assigned to the study.

III. Technician's Responsibilities Related to Investigational Drugs

A. Assists in the development of detailed procedures for preparation, dispensing, and distribution of investigational drugs.

B. Assists in developing and maintaining established record-keeping systems for protocols, study subjects, drug inventory, and preparation and dispensing of investigational drugs.

C. Assists in establishing and maintaining standards to ensure the quality, proper storage, and safe use of investigational drugs.

D. Maintains adequate inventory levels for each study using established ordering systems and inventory control procedures. Removes and disposes of expired stock from investigational studies according to protocol guidelines or departmental policy.

E. Makes accurate entries into protocol report forms and established record-keeping systems.

F. Assists the IDS pharmacist in the preparation of investigational drugs.

IV. Technician's Role in Collecting and Communicating Data Related to Investigational Drugs

A. Reconciles each investigational drug order with the corresponding protocol and study subject.

B. Communicates with study monitors and other associated personnel to verify unique administration time schedules.

C. Contacts study coordinators when doses of investigational drugs are returned to the pharmacy unused.

D. Provides drug information materials or monograph to nurses when the first dose of an investigational drug is dispensed. These materials should be kept with the patient's medication administration record.

E. Assists in the development of statistical reports and activity summaries on a monthly basis. Assists with monthly audits to ensure that IDS policies and procedures are met. May assist with quality assurance procedures as needed.

F. Prepares for audits of inventory, drug-dispensing records, and files by investigators or study sponsors.

G. Assists the IDS pharmacist in various activities as needed. Examples include:
   1. Reviewing protocols, materials, and services required to fulfill the study objectives

   2. Meeting with investigators, study monitors, and others to coordinate study logistics

   3. Assisting with budget preparation for investigational drug studies

   4. Submitting monthly or periodic charges for use of pharmaceutical services to billing department and maintaining a record of all charges for each study

V. Chapter Summary

A. Technicians must be knowledgeable about policies, procedures, and specific protocols for handling, preparing, and dispensing investigational drugs. Detailed documentation must be accurate and complete.

B. The technician's role in collecting and communicating data related to investigational drugs may include meeting with study monitors, providing drug information to other health care workers, and evaluating procedures required to fulfill the study objectives.

C. Technicians may be called upon to assist the IDS pharmacist in coordinating study logistics and preparation of budgets for selected studies.

VI. Questions for Discussion

A. List five parameters that might be included in a protocol for an investigational drug.

B. Why do investigational drugs require specific and extensive protocols?

C. Discuss four aspects to consider when handling and processing investigational drugs.

D. Name six technician responsibilities related to investigational drug studies.

E. Why is the technician's role important in collecting and communicating data on investigational drugs?

VII. Sample Questions

A. Why are investigational drugs tested in the community?

1. To determine efficacy of investigational drugs using a larger study group than clinical trials allow

2. To ensure that they are effective and safe in the general population

3. To study more thoroughly specific patient populations with particular diseases

4. May help patients who have failed other therapies to determine whether the investigational drug or regimen is better than the previous therapies

5. All of the above reasons

B. Protocols and procedures regarding investigational drugs:

1. Are developed by the principal investigator independently

2. Describe the procedures for preparation and storage

3. Provide information on the proper dosage and monitoring parameters for patients enrolled in the study

4. All of the above apply

5. Only 2 and 3 apply

C. Why is scheduling important when dispensing investigational drugs?

1. Stability may be limited.

2. The principal investigator may offer therapy at unusual times to meet the needs of particular patients.

3. Scheduling follows protocols to achieve maximum patient response to therapy.

4. Record-keeping helps ensure that schedules are met and that the patient receives the medication at the appropriate times.

5. All of the above are correct.

D. True or false?

1. Investigational drugs may be used indiscriminately by physicians to treat patients who do not respond to other therapies.

2. Record-keeping procedures for investigational drugs are determined only by the principal investigators.

3. Technicians may provide information about the investigational drug to nurses caring for patients in the study.

4. Investigational drugs should be labeled only with exactly the same information as other drugs (e.g., name, strength, administration, expiration date).

5. Technicians must be knowledgeable about the drugs being studied and be familiar with appropriate documentation regarding investigational drugs.

6. The drug monograph must be provided to the nursing staff no sooner than delivery of the second dose of the drug being studied.

E. Inventory levels for investigational drugs are affected by:

1. Stability

2. Protocol guidelines

3. Record-keeping procedures

4. All of the above

5. 1 and 2 only

Answers appear on page 144.

Notes:

Chapter Seven

Collecting and Communicating Data on Restricted Drug Distribution Programs
Procedures for Restricted Drug Distribution Programs

I. Key Terms and Concepts

A. Restricted drugs (RD)
   1. Drugs that are rarely used, have limited therapeutic options, and small patient populations. Registration allows the monitoring of efficacy and safety of drugs that have limited use because of side effects and unintended consequences. The technician assists the pharmacist in dispensing and recording the distribution of these agents. All of these drugs are approved for specific indications but require postmarketing restrictions because of serious side effects.

II. Examples of Restricted Drugs

A. Thalidomide (Thalomid®)
   1. Thalidomide is approved for acute treatment, maintenance therapy, and preventive therapy of skin manifestations related to moderate to severe erythema nodosum leprosum (ENL).

   2. Thalidomide is associated with teratogenicity, usually resulting in limb deformities of fetuses exposed in utero. Women of childbearing age and capability are warned not to use or handle thalidomide.

   3. S.T.E.P.S.® is a restricted distribution program developed by Celgene Corporation that requires:
      a. Product labeling that includes information about the risks of taking thalidomide and a boxed warning to highlight side effects and severe risks.

      b. Registration of all prescribers, patients, and pharmacists, and pharmacies who prescribe, receive, and dispense thalidomide.

      c. Pregnancy testing and patient consent form, brochure, and videotape that describe side effect warnings about birth defects and fetal abnormalities.

      d. Requirement for women of childbearing potential to have a pregnancy test within 24 hours prior to taking thalidomide and to take pregnancy tests for the first 4 weeks and 28 days thereafter. They also must use at least one highly effective birth control method.

      e. Limitation of quantity to a 28-day supply provided in blister packs with safety information on the packs.

    f. Prohibition of telephone prescriptions and automatic refills.

    g. Quality assurance activities of S.T.E.P.S.® program that provide ongoing evaluation of the program.

    h. Physicians obtain authorization after completing a phone survey. An authorization number is placed on the prescription and sent to the Interactive Voice Response (IVR) system. Without the authorization number, the drug may not be dispensed. The pharmacist calls the IVR system, enters the authorization number, activates the prescription, and receives authorization to dispense the prescription.

B. Isotretinoin products (Accutane®, Amnesteem®, Claravis®, Sotret®)
1. Isotretinoin is approved to treat severe, disfiguring nodular acne and certain skin diseases when other therapies have failed.

2. Like thalidomide, isotretinoin is associated with adverse effects on fetal development and must not be used in women who are able to bear children.
    a. The System to Manage Accutane Related Teratogenicity (SMART) program is a risk-management program that includes:
        (1) Self-certification program of physicians who plan to prescribe isotretinoin

        (2) Patient agreement

        (3) FDA-approved medication guide

        (4) Dispensing requirements:
            (a) No more than a 30-day supply

            (b) Presence of a yellow prescribing program sticker for both male and female patients

            (c) Prescription written within previous 7 days; no telephone or computerized prescriptions (except iPLEDGE program prescriptions)

            (d) Patient given medication guide each time isotretinoin is dispensed

C. Clozapine (Clozaril®)
1. Clozapine is indicated for the treatment of severe schizophrenia in patients who have failed standard therapy.

2. Clozapine may cause life-threatening side effects including agranulocytosis, seizures, myocarditis, other adverse cardiovascular and respiratory effects, and increased mortality in geriatric patients with dementia-related psychosis.

3. Registration and monitoring procedures include the following:
    a. Patients must be registered with the IVAX Pharmaceuticals Clozapine Patient Registration or the Clozaril National Registry (CNR) prior to dispensing IVAX clozapine or Clozaril® (Novartis).

    b. A current and acceptable white blood cell (WBC) count is required.

    c. A 1- to 2-week supply may be dispensed when a patient meets the requirements and is registered.

    d. White blood cell monitoring is routinely conducted during therapy.

D. Alosetron (Lotronex™)
1. Alosetron is used for the treatment of women with severe, diarrhea-prominent irritable bowel syndrome (IBS) who have failed to respond to conventional therapy.

2. Alosetron was withdrawn from the market following postmarketing reports of severe and sometimes life-threatening ischemic colitis and complications of constipation, including death.

3. Distribution program. Alosetron was reintroduced into the market in 2002, subject to a risk management program called the Prescribing Program for LOTRONEX™ that requires:
    a. Enrollment and self-certification of physicians

    b. Patient-physician agreement form

    c. Written prescriptions only

    d. Prescribing program sticker on all written prescriptions

    e. Medication guide provided with every dispensed prescription

E. Other restricted drugs
1. Bosentan (Tracleer®)

2. Dofetilide (Tikosyn®)

3. Gefitinib (Iressa®)

III. Chapter Summary

Pharmacy technicians should be aware that new uses are discovered for older drugs that were once deemed too dangerous because of severe adverse reactions. Sometimes new drugs that had acceptable side effects in clinical studies are later found to have serious adverse effects when used in a larger group of patients. These drugs gain "restricted" status because they provide the most effective therapy for particular patients when certain conditions are met. Patients receiving restricted drugs must qualify under strict protocols and must be monitored closely.

IV. Questions for Discussion

A. With all the potential adverse effects, why are restricted drugs still on the market?

B. When handling thalidomide tablets, what is the primary concern facing the technician, pharmacist, or nurse?

C. When a technician receives a prescription for thalidomide, how does he or she know whether or not it is approved under restricted drug guidelines?

D. Why was the restricted drug program created?

V. Sample Questions

A. What must *always* be confirmed by the pharmacy technician or pharmacist before thalidomide is dispensed?

　　1. The patient's diagnosis

　　2. The number of refills assigned on the basis of duration of therapy

　　3. Verification of the authorization number

　　4. Any prior use of thalidomide by patient

　　5. All of the above

B. Which statement is not true about criteria that must be met before a patient may receive clozapine?

　　1. Patients must be registered with IVAX Pharmaceuticals.

　　2. White blood cell count must be determined and monitored.

　　3. Patients may receive more than a 1–2 week supply if they meet the requirements and are registered with IVAX Pharmaceuticals.

　　4. Patients who have severe schizophrenia unresponsive to standard therapy are candidates for clozapine therapy.

　　5. All of the above statements are true.

C. True or false?

1. Thalidomide use is strictly prohibited in women of childbearing age.

2. Isotretinoin is commonly used to treat severe, disfiguring acne unresponsive to standard therapy, especially in young women.

3. Patients receiving restricted drugs are monitored for only 1 year. Thereafter, they may receive the drug without following restricted drug protocols.

4. The program S.T.E.P.S.® developed by Celgene Corporation requires that pregnancy testing be conducted before authorizing therapy with thalidomide.

5. IVAX Pharmaceuticals has set up a registration procedure for patients eligible to receive clozapine.

D. Alosetron is restricted for use in only:

1. IBS patients who have been stabilized on other medications

2. IBS patients who are experiencing constipation

3. Patients with severe, nodular acne lesions

4. Women with severe diarrhea-prominent IBS

5. None of the above

Answers appear on page 144.

Notes:

Section IV

Participating in the Administration and Management of Pharmacy Practice

Includes activities related to the administrative processes for the pharmacy practice site, including operations, human resources, facilities and equipment, and information systems

Chapter Eight

Operations

I. Coordinating Communications Throughout the Practice Site and/or Service Area

   A. Intradepartmental/interdepartmental communications
      1. Verbal communication
         a. Phone calls
            (1) Phone calls may be addressed directly or routed to the appropriate recipient. Some examples include:
               (a) Routing to pharmacist when physician is calling

               (b) Routing to pharmacist when registered nurse is calling with a new prescription or medication order

               (c) Routing to other appropriate recipient (e.g., other technicians, pharmacy directors, administrators), depending on the specific type of information (e.g., change in intravenous orders, patient discharge) to be communicated

               (d) Accepting calls from physicians or their representatives to authorize refills

         b. Interpersonal communication
            (1) Accepting, communicating, and transmitting messages and information to, and from, those involved

      2. Written communication
         a. Routing faxes to appropriate recipients

         b. Processing prescriptions and medication orders

         c. Routing other written communications

   B. Participating in meetings
      1. Obtaining feedback regarding the performance of the practice site and/or service area

II. Monitoring the Practice Site and/or Service Area for Compliance with Federal, State, and Local Laws, Regulations, and Professional Standards

III. Implementing and Monitoring Policies and Procedures for Environmental Safety

A. Sanitation management

B. Hazardous waste handling (e.g., needles)

C. Infection control (e.g., protective clothing)

IV. Performing and Recording Routine Sanitation, Maintenance, and Calibration of Equipment

A. Equipment must be cleaned, sanitized, maintained, and calibrated at regularly scheduled intervals (or more often as necessary) to prevent contamination and to ensure proper performance.

B. Policies and procedures established for the cleaning and maintenance of equipment must be followed.

C. Records should be kept of equipment cleaning, maintenance, and inspection.

V. Maintaining a Computer-Based Information System

A. Computer systems are used for:

1. Processing prescriptions and medication orders

2. Inventory control

3. Controlled-substances tracking

4. Updating drug prices

5. Administrative functions
   a. Workload and productivity tracking

   b. Drug utilization review

   c. Third-party authorization, billing, and reconciliation

VI. Maintaining Software for Computerized Systems

    A. Automated dispensing technology

    B. Point-of-care drug dispensing cabinets

VII. Personnel Functions

    A. Performing or contributing to employee evaluations

    B. Establishing, implementing, and monitoring policies and procedures

VIII. Chapter Summary

    A. Technicians should be knowledgeable about the activities, policies, and procedures related to the administrative processes for the pharmacy practice site, including how and when to perform routine maintenance and calibration of equipment, monitoring the practice site for compliance with regulations and professional standards, and maintaining the pharmacy's information systems.

IX. Questions for Discussion

    A. Discuss methods for coordinating communications throughout the practice site and/or service area.

    B. Describe the various functions that can be managed and tracked using computer-based information systems.

X. Sample Questions

    A. The pharmacy technician's role includes monitoring which of the following:

        1. Compliance with federal, state, and local laws

        2. Compliance with regulations related to the handling of controlled substances

        3. Policies and procedures for environmental safety

        4. Quality control procedures used in the pharmacy

        5. All of the above answers are included in the technician's responsibilities.

B. Which of the following instruments should be routinely *calibrated*?

1. Prescription balance

2. Laminar airflow hood

3. Graduated cylinder

4. Mortar and pestle

5. All of the above

Answers appear on page 144.

Notes:

Section V

Pharmaceutical Calculations

Includes mathematical calculations related to the pharmacy practice site, including calculation of doses and injection flow rates, conversions between units of measurement, percentage preparations, reduction and enlargement of formulas, and determination of charges for prescriptions and medication orders

Chapter Nine

Fractions, Decimals, and Roman Numerals

I. Fractions

A. Components of fractions
   1. Example: 5/8
      Numerator   5
      Fraction line —
      Denominator   8

B. Types of common fractions
   1. Proper fractions
      a. Proper fractions are fractions with a smaller numerator than denominator.
         (1) Example: 5/8

   2. Improper fractions
      a. Improper fractions are fractions with a larger numerator than denominator.
         (1) Example: 8/5

      b. Improper fractions should be reduced to a mixed number.
         (1) Example: 8/5 should be reduced to 1 3/5

   3. Simple fractions
      a. Simple fractions are proper fractions reduced to lowest terms.
         (1) Example: 15/24 = 5/8

   4. Complex fractions
      a. Complex fractions are "fractions of fractions," where both the numerator and denominator are fractions.
         (1) Example: $\dfrac{5/8}{1/2}$

C. Reducing fractions to lowest terms
   1. In reducing fractions, the fraction maintains its value but changes its form. Reduction of a fraction to lowest terms is accomplished by dividing both the numerator and denominator by the largest multiple that is common to both terms.

    a. Example: 15/24 is reduced to 5/8 by dividing both numerator and denominator by 3:

$$\frac{15 \div 3 \; = \; 5}{24 \div 3 \; = \; 8}$$

D. Five rules for calculating with fractions
    1. Understand the impact of multiplying or dividing the numerator and/or denominator by a whole number.
        Example: 4/8

$$\frac{4 \times 2}{8} = \frac{8}{8} = 1 \qquad\qquad \frac{4}{8 \times 2} = \frac{4}{16} = \frac{1}{4}$$

$$\frac{4 \div 2}{8} = \frac{2}{8} = \frac{1}{4} \qquad\qquad \frac{4}{8 \div 2} = \frac{4}{4} = 1$$

    2. Convert mixed numbers or whole numbers to improper fractions before performing calculations with other fractions.
        a. Example: 2 7/8 = 23/8

    3. When adding or subtracting fractions, make sure all fractions have a common denominator (i.e., a number into which all denominators may be divided an even number of times).
        a. Example: 3/4, 5/8, 1/2 may be written as 6/8, 5/8, 4/8

    4. Convert answers that are improper fractions back to whole numbers or mixed numbers.
        a. Example: 15/3 = 5

    5. Convert answers to lowest terms
        a. Example: 16/32 = 8/16 = 4/8 = 2/4 = 1/2

E. Adding and subtracting fractions
    1. All fractions must first be converted so that they have a common denominator. The numerators are then added or subtracted.
        a. Example: 1/2 + 5/6 + 3/8 = 12/24 + 20/24 + 9/24 = 41/24 = 1 17/24

        b. Example: 13/32 – 3/8 = 13/32 – 12/32 = 1/32

F. Multiplying fractions
    1. Unlike addition and subtraction, multiplication of fractions does not require common denominators. Multiply numerators by numerators and denominators by denominators.
        a. Example: 9 2/7 × 3/4 = 65/7 × 3/4 = 195/28 = 6 27/28

G. Dividing fractions
    1. Invert the divisor and multiply the fractions.
        a. Example: $11/12 \div 1/6 = 11/12 \times 6/1 = 66/12 = 5\ 1/2$

        b. Example: $10\ 3/5 \div 2\ 1/10 = 53/5 \div 21/10 = 53/5 \times 10/21 = 530/105 = 5\ 5/105 = 5\ 1/21$

II. Decimals

A. Converting decimals to fractions
    1. Decimal fractions are fractions with denominators of 10 and/or multiples of 10.
        a. A decimal number with one digit to the right of the decimal point is expressed in "tenths."
            (1) Example: $0.7 = 7/10$

        b. A decimal number with two digits to the right of the decimal point is expressed as "hundredths."
            (1) Example: $0.27 = 27/100$

        c. Follow the same rule as more digits are added to the right of the decimal point.
            (1) Example: $0.0365 = 365/10,000$

B. Converting fractions to decimals
    1. To convert common fractions to decimal fractions, divide the numerator by the denominator.
        a. Example: $3/4 = 0.75$

        b. Example: $1\ 5/8 = 13/8 = 1.625$

C. Adding, subtracting, multiplying, and dividing decimals
    1. When adding, subtracting, multiplying, and dividing decimals and common fractions, convert all terms to the same system before performing the calculation.
        a. Example: $25/100 + 1.005 = 0.25 + 1.005 = 1.255$

III. Roman Numerals

A. Primary Roman numeral units
    SS = 1/2
    I or i = 1
    V = 5
    X = 10
    L = 50
    C = 100
    D = 500
    M = 1000

B. Eight rules for use of Roman numerals
1. When a numeral is repeated, its value is repeated.
   a. Example: XX = 10 + 10 = 20

2. A numeral may not be repeated more than three times.
   a. Example: XL = 40 not XXXX

3. V, L, and D are never repeated. VV is incorrect.

4. When a smaller numeral is placed before a larger numeral, it is subtracted from the larger numeral.
   a. Example: XC = 100 – 10 = 90

5. When a smaller numeral is placed after a larger numeral, it is added to the larger numeral.
   a. Example: CX = 100 + 10 = 110

6. V, L, and D are never subtracted. VX is incorrect.

7. Never subtract more than one numeral.
   a. Example: VIII = 8 not IIX

8. Use I before V and X (only the next two highest numerals). The same is true for X and C (X before L and C; C before D and M).

IV. Sample Questions

A. Reduce the following fractions to lowest terms:
1. 10/75 = _____
2. 8/16 = _____
3. 3/15 = _____
4. 60/186 = _____

B. Convert the following numbers to improper fractions:
1. 5 = _____
2. 3 2/3 = _____

C. Convert the following groups of fractions into groups of fractions with common denominators:
1. 15/32, 3/16, 7/64 = _____, _____, _____
2. 3/4, 7/8, 5/12 = _____, _____, _____

D. Convert 15/4 into a whole or mixed number: 15/4 = _____

E. 3/4 + 1 1/8 = _____

F. 7 5/8 – 1 1/3 = _____

G. $1\ 3/4 \times 3 =$ _____

H. $1/2 \div 5 =$ _____

I. $3/16 \div 1\ 1/2 =$ _____

J. Convert the following decimal numbers to fractions:
1. $0.07 =$ _____
2. $0.077 =$ _____
3. $5.0125 =$ _____

K. Convert the following fractions to decimal numbers:
1. $3/8 =$ _____
2. $2\ 7/13 =$ _____

L. Perform the following calculations:
1. $3.75 - 1/2 =$ _____
2. $3/4 \times 2.5 =$ _____
3. $2\ 3/8 \div 0.5 =$ _____

M. Express the following numbers as roman numerals:
1. $29 =$ _____
2. $47 =$ _____
3. $86 =$ _____
4. $1154 =$ _____

N. Express the following roman numerals as Arabic numerals:
1. LXXVIII = _____
2. CXIII = _____
3. XCIV = _____
4. MCMLXI = _____

O. How many 0.0125 grain (gr.) doses can be made from 3/8 gr. of a drug?

P. How many ounces of boric acid would be left in an 8-oz. bottle if you dispensed 2 prescriptions each containing 1 1/4 oz. of boric acid and 3 additional prescriptions each containing 1.75 oz. from the bottle?

Q. How many 1/40 gr. tablets would provide 1/200 gr. of a drug?

R. How many 1/400 gr. nitroglycerin tablets would provide 1/150 gr. of nitroglycerin?

S. If 10 patients each receive XLIV mg of a drug, how many total milligrams (in Roman numerals) would all the patients receive?

T. How much would a compounded ointment weigh if it contained the following weights of various drugs and vehicles: IX grams, VI grams, and LX grams?

U. How many pounds of a chemical are remaining if a manufacturer has DXV pounds of the chemical and uses LXVI pounds to manufacture a bulk powder?

V. A capsule contains CDXLV milligrams of a drug. How many milligrams would be in 20 capsules?

W. Express the total weight in Roman numerals of 4 applications of an eye ointment if each application weighs 251 mg.

X. How many prescriptions (in Roman numerals) are filled in a pharmacy over 4 days if the pharmacy averages CXX prescriptions daily?

Y. 1. How many pounds of sulfur powder does a pharmacy have on hand if the pharmacy has 3 containers each containing 3/8 lb. of sulfur?

    2. How much sulfur would remain if you gave 3/16 lb. of sulfur to another pharmacy?

Z. A hospitalized patient received 4 doses of 1/150 gr. nitroglycerin tablets in 1 day. How many grains of nitroglycerin did the patient receive? *(Express answer as a decimal fraction.)*

AA. 1. A 120-ml bottle of children's antihistamine syrup contains 24 tsp. doses. How many milliliters must be in a dose?

     2. How many doses would be in the bottle if a young child receives 3/4 tsp. of the syrup per dose?

BB. How many milligrams of aspirin would be in XXIV tablets if each tablet contains 325 mg of aspirin?

CC. 1. A pharmacy technician has 200 g of Drug B on hand. How much will be required to fill 100 capsules each containing 1 1/8 g of Drug B?

2. How many grams of Drug B remain after filling the capsules?

DD. If the average pharmacy technician can prepare CIX prescriptions daily, how many technicians would be required to prepare MDCXXXV prescriptions?

EE. How many 0.004 g doses can be made from 3/4 g of a drug?

Answers appear on pages 144–145.

Notes:

Chapter Ten

Calculating Percentage and Ratio Strength

I. Percentage

A. Percent and its corresponding sign (%) mean "parts in one hundred."
   1. Example: 40% may also be expressed as:
      a. 40 parts in a 100

      b. 40/100

      c. 0.40

      d. 2/5 (40/100 = 4/10 = 2/5)

B. Converting percents to decimals
   1. To change percents to decimals, remove the percent sign and move the decimal two places to the left.
      a. Examples: 58% = 58/100 or 0.58   72% = 72/100 or 0.72

C. Converting decimals and fractions to percents
   1. Converting a decimal to a percent
      a. To convert a decimal to a percent, move the decimal two places to the right and add the percent sign.
         (1) Example: 0.17 = 17%

D. Percent expressed as a ratio
   1. A ratio is the relationship or comparison of two like quantities.
      a. Example: 1/2 expressed as a ratio would be 1:2 or "one part in two parts." This can also be expressed as:
         (1) a decimal (0.5)

         (2) a percent (50%)

2. Converting a fraction to a percent
   a. To convert a fraction to a percent, reduce the fraction to a decimal, then move the decimal two places to the right, and add the percent sign.
      (1) Example: $1/2 = 0.50 = 50\%$

II. Ratio and Proportion

A. Proportion
   1. A proportion is the expression of the equality of two ratios or fractions. Most pharmacy calculations can be done by using the principles of ratio and proportion.

B. Basic algebraic expression
   1. The simplest algebraic form for a ratio and proportion is: $A/B = C/D$, or $A{:}B = C{:}D$

C. Solving for an unknown
   1. By setting two equal ratios together, you may easily solve for an unknown if you know three terms of a proportion.
      a. Example: $3/5 = x/15$
         This can be restated as, "if there are 3 parts in 5 parts, then there are x parts in 15 parts."
         Cross multiply to get: $5(x) = 45$
         Rearrange the equation to: $(x) = 45/5$
         Divide to get the solution: $x = 45/5 = 9$
         Therefore, $3/5 = 9/15$, or "3 parts in 5 parts is equivalent to 9 parts in every 15 parts."

III. Sample Questions

A. Convert the following:

   1. $72\% = 72/100 = 0.\underline{\hspace{1cm}}$

   2. $0.35 = 35\% = \underline{\hspace{1cm}}/100 = 7/\underline{\hspace{1cm}}$

   3. $25\% = 25/100 = \underline{\hspace{1cm}}{:}100$

   4. $0.182 = \underline{\hspace{1cm}}\%$

   5. $3/8 = 0.\underline{\hspace{1cm}} = \underline{\hspace{1cm}}\%$

B. Using the principles of ratio and proportion, solve the following:

   1. If 10 lb. of drug cost $200, what would 2 lb. cost?

2. How many pounds could you buy for $25?

3. What would 10 oz. cost (16 oz. per 1 lb.)?

C. A formula for 1000 tablets contains 11.5 g of an antihistamine. How many grams of the antihistamine should be used to prepare 475 tablets?

D. A cough syrup contains 5 mg of a drug in each 15 ml dose.
How many milligrams of drug would be contained in a 480 ml bottle of syrup?

E. If 2 tablets contain 650 mg of acetaminophen, how many milligrams would be contained in a bottle of 100 tablets?

F. If 7 tablets contain 35 mg of diazepam, how many tablets would contain 1500 mg?

G. If a patient pays $0.58 per tablet for 90 tablets, how much does the entire prescription cost?

H. How many grams of codeine sulfate would be required to prepare 20 capsules, each containing 0.0325 g of codeine sulfate?

I. How much would 100 lb. of a chemical cost if 385 lb. cost $795?

J. How many kilograms would a 173-lb. patient weigh if there are 2.2 lb. in every kilogram?

K. If a penicillin solution contains 6 million units of penicillin in 10 ml, how many units would be contained in a 0.5 ml dose?

L. If a patient receives 5 ml of intravenous fluid per minute, how much fluid would the patient receive each hour?

M. How many milligrams of amoxicillin would a patient receive in 1 week if the patient receives 750 mg each day?

N. If a syringe contains 28 mg of drug in 3 ml, how many milligrams of the drug would a patient receive if 1.2 ml is administered?

O. If a 480 ml bottle of 10% potassium chloride solution contains 10 g of potassium chloride in every 100 ml of solution, how much potassium chloride will a patient receive from a 15 ml dose of the solution?

P. In the previous question, how much would the bottle of potassium chloride cost if the 15 ml dose cost $0.28?

Q. 1. If 12 prescription bottles cost $1.80, how much would 9 bottles cost?

   2. How much would a case containing 10 dozen bottles cost?

R. 1. If a technician fills 1 prescription every 270 seconds, how many minutes would it take to fill a single prescription?

   2. How many prescriptions can the technician fill in a 7.5-hour workday?

S. 1. A tablet contains 5 mg of an active ingredient. How many tablets should be dispensed for 1 month (*assume 30 days*) of therapy if the patient receives 1 tablet t.i.d.?

   2. How many milligrams of the drug will the patient receive in 1 month?

T. 1. A 454 g jar of ointment contains 4.54 g of hydrocortisone. What is the decimal fraction of hydrocortisone in the ointment?

   2. What is the percent strength of this ointment?

U. A cream is labeled 20% strength. Express this value as a ratio strength.

V. 1. If 6 oz. of a drug cost $88, how much would 1/4 oz. cost?

    2. How much of the drug can be purchased for $1?

W. 1. If 100 capsules contain 3/8 g of an active ingredient, how many grams will 50 capsules contain (*express answer as a common fraction*)?

    2. Express the previous answer as a percent of a gram.

Answers appear on pages 145–146.

Notes:

Chapter Eleven

Pharmaceutical Systems of Measurement

I. Metric System

A. Primary units (subdivided by multiples of 10)
   1. Length: meter (m)

   2. Volume: liter (L or l)

   3. Weight: gram (g)

B. Common prefixes
   1. "Increasing" prefix
      a. "Kilo-" (1000) is the most common increasing prefix.
         (1) Example: 1 kilogram (kg) = 1000 g

   2. "Decreasing" prefixes
      a. "Milli-" (1/1000)
         (1) Example: 1 milligram (mg) = 0.001 g (1/1000 g)

         (2) Example: 1 g = 1000 mg

      b. "Micro-" (1/1,000,000)
         (1) Example: 1 microgram (mcg or μg) = 0.000001 g

         (2) Example: 1 g = 1,000,000 mcg

II. Common Conversions Between Systems

A. "Rounded-off" conversion factors
   1. Weight
      a. 1 gram (g) = 15.4 grains (gr.)

      b. 1 grain (gr.) = 65 milligrams (mg)

      c. 1 pound (lb.) = 454 grams (g)

    d. 1 kilogram (kg) = 2.2 pounds (lb.)

    e. 1 ounce (oz.) = 28.4 grams (g)

    f. 1 ounce (oz.) = 437.5 grains (gr.)

    g. 1 pound (lb.) = 16 ounces (oz.)

2. Volume
    a. 1 fluid ounce = 30 milliliters (ml)

    b. 1 pint = 16 fluid ounces = 480 milliliters
       (*Note:* Sometimes the label on a pint bottle will read 473 ml instead of 480 ml.
       A fluid ounce actually contains 29.57 ml but is frequently rounded to 30 ml.)

    c. 1 gallon = 4 quarts = 8 pints = 128 fluid ounces = 3840 milliliters

3. Length
    a. 1 inch = 2.54 cm

III. Temperature Conversions

A. Converting degrees centigrade to degrees Fahrenheit
    1. $°F = 32 + 9/5°C$
       a. Example: 25°C
          $32 + 9/5 (25) = 77°F$

B. Converting degrees Fahrenheit to degrees centigrade
    1. $°C = 5/9 (°F − 32)$
       a. Example: 32°F
          $5/9 (32 − 32) = 0°C$

IV. Sample Questions

A. Convert the following metric system units:

    1. 225 kilometers = _____ m

    2. 525 g = _____ kg

    3. 5 g = _____ mg = _____ mcg

    4. 350 ml = _____ L

B. Calculate the following conversions:

   1. 16 fluid oz. = 1 pt. = _____ ml

   2. 2 pt. = 1 qt. = _____ fluid oz.

   3. 4 qt. = 1 gal. = _____ pt. = _____ fluid oz.

C. Solve the following conversions:

   1. 16 oz. = 1 lb. = _____ gr.

   2. 3 inches = _____ cm

D. Using the rounded-off conversion factor for weight, fill in the blanks:

   1. 1 gr. = _____ g = _____ mg

   2. 1 oz. = _____ gr.= _____ g

   3. 1 lb. = _____ oz. = _____ g = _____ gr. = _____ kg

   4. 1 kg = _____ lb.

E. Using the rounded-off conversion factor for volume, fill in the blanks:

   1. 1 pt. = _____ fluid oz. = _____ ml

   2. 1 gal. = _____ fluid oz. = _____ ml = _____ L

F. Convert 20°C to degrees Fahrenheit.

G. Convert 212°F to degrees centigrade.

H. How many 325 mg aspirin tablets can be prepared from 1/2 kg of aspirin?

I. How many kilograms would a 246-lb. patient weigh?

J. A 10 ml vial contains 40 mg of a drug. How many micrograms would be administered by injection of 2 ml of the drug?

K. If a physician orders 10 g of drug per liter, how many grains would be in 250 ml?

L. 1. A pharmacy purchases 1.8 lb. of an antibiotic powder for compounding. How many ounces were purchased?

   2. How much did the bulk powder cost if 1 oz. costs $8.75?

   3. How much would 3/4 oz. cost?

M. 1. How many 4 fluid oz. bottles can be filled from 3 gal. of syrup?

   2. How much would 1 bottle cost if the syrup sells for $40 per gallon?

N. 1. How many kilograms of a drug would be needed to manufacture 800,000 tablets, each containing 15 mg of the drug?

   2. Express the previous answer in pounds.

   3. Express the previous answer in ounces.

   4. How much would the total amount of drug in the previous question cost if 1 oz. sells for $14.85?

O. 1. A patient weights 185 lb., but a drug is dosed on the basis of the patient's weight in kilograms. How many kilograms does the patient weigh?

   2. How much of a drug should this patient receive if the recommended dose is 3 mg/kg of body weight?

P. The temperature last January in Moscow was –58°F. Express this temperature in degrees centigrade.

Q. A certain plastic cracks at –15°C. Express this temperature in degrees Fahrenheit.

Answers appear on pages 146–147.

Notes:

Chapter Twelve

Dosage Calculations

I. Basic Principles in Dosing

A. Key terms and concepts
   1. Dose
      a. The quantity of a drug taken by a patient is known as the dose. The dose may be expressed as a "daily" dose, "single" dose, or even a "total" dose, which refers to the entire quantity of the drug taken throughout therapy. Daily doses may be given once daily, which is a single dose, or may be divided throughout the day.

   2. Dosage regimen
      a. A dosage regimen refers to the schedule of medication administration (e.g., every 4 hours, 3 times a day, at bedtime).

B. Doses vary tremendously because of differences in drug potency; routes of administration; the patient's age, weight, kidney, and liver functions, etc. Many factors can enter into establishing a correct dose, and many dispensing errors are related to administering the wrong dose. Pharmacy technicians can contribute to patient care by being familiar with appropriate doses of medications and by being able to calculate doses to check questionable orders.

II. Manufacturer's Recommended Dose

A. Manufacturers of medications establish the normal doses of drugs through research. This information can be obtained from numerous sources including package inserts, *Physician's Desk Reference (PDR)*, *USP DI*, *Facts and Comparisons*, and other sources. These doses are usually listed as milligrams or milliliters per kilogram (or pound) of body weight. The calculation of doses can usually be performed by simply using the principles of ratio and proportion.

   1. Example: The dose of a drug is 10 mg per kg of body weight. How much would you give a 220-lb. man?
      a. Step 1: 2.2 lb./1 kg = 220 lb./x
         x = 100 kg of body weight

      b. Step 2: 10 mg drug/1 kg = x/100 kg
         x = 1000 mg = 1 g of drug

III. Household Equivalents

A. Household equivalents are measurements frequently used in dosing. They are referred to as "household equivalents" because they are measures frequently found in homes (teaspoons, pints, tablespoons, etc.).

   1. 1 teaspoonful (tsp.) = 5 ml

   2. 1 tablespoonful (tbsp.) = 15 ml

   3. 1 fluid ounce = 30 ml

IV. Flow Rate Calculations

A. Flow rate calculations are normally used for intravenous solutions and can be done by "multiple" ratio and proportion calculations.

   1. Example: If an intravenous order is for 500 ml of D5NS (5% dextrose in 0.9% sodium chloride) to be given over 4 hours (240 minutes), and the IV set delivers 15 drops (gtt.) per milliliter, what would be the flow rate?

   Step 1: $\dfrac{15 \text{ gtt.}}{1 \text{ ml}} = \dfrac{x}{50 \text{ ml}}$ x = 7500 total drops (gtt.)

   Step 2: $\dfrac{7500 \text{ gtt.}}{240 \text{ min.}} = \dfrac{x}{1 \text{ min.}}$ x = 31 gtt./min.

Note: Another method for calculating flow rates is by using the following formula:

$$\frac{(\text{ml/hr.}) \ (\text{gtt./ml})}{60 \text{ min./hr.}} = \text{ flow rate in gtt./min.}$$

Using the above example:

$$\frac{(500 \text{ ml/4 hr.}) \ (15 \text{ gtt./ml})}{60 \text{ min./hr.}} = 31 \text{ gtt./min.}$$

V. Body Surface Area

A. Dosing by a patient's body surface area (BSA) is based on the individual's volume rather than weight. This method is used frequently with patients who are receiving chemotherapy and sometimes with children. BSA is measured in square meters (m^2), and most of the dosing will be in milligrams per square meter (mg/m^2).

1. BSA can be determined by finding out a patient's height and weight, and then using a nomogram (see page 101).

   a. Five steps to determine a patient's BSA using a nomogram
      (1) Select the appropriate nomogram (i.e., adult or child).

      (2) Place a dot on the value for the patient's height (left vertical axis).

      (3) Place a dot on the value for the patient's weight (right vertical axis).

      (4) Connect the dots in steps 2 and 3 with a straight edge.

      (5) Read the patient's BSA located on the center vertical axis at the point where it is intersected by the line drawn in step 4.

      Example: What is the BSA for a 52-year-old man who is 170 cm tall and weighs 70 kg?

      Answer: BSA = 1.8 m^2

      Solution: Using the adult nomogram, place a dot on the left vertical axis at 170 cm and a dot on the right vertical axis at 70 kg. Connect the dots using a straight edge, and read the patient's BSA on the center vertical axis at the point where it is intersected by the straight line.

VI. Chemotherapy Dosing

A. BSA is frequently used for dosing chemotherapeutic drugs for cancer patients. There are many safety considerations that must be taken into account in prescribing, compounding, and administering antineoplastic drugs. Correct dosing is a critical concern. Dosing chemotherapeutic drugs is frequently done by establishing the patient's BSA (see previous section) and then determining the dose by the ratio and proportion method.

Example: How many milligrams of paclitaxel would a 42-year-old, 131-lb., 65-inch-tall female patient receive if the intravenous adult dose for breast carcinoma is 175 mg per square meter of BSA repeated every 21 days?

Step 1: Use adult nomogram to determine the BSA: 1.65 m^2

Step 2: Determine dose by ratio and proportion method:
175 mg/m^2 = x/1.65 m^2
x = 289 mg

VII. Sample Questions

A. Solve the following using the principles of ratio and proportion:

1. 1 tbsp.= 15 ml = _____ tsp.

2. 1 fluid oz. = 30 ml = _____ tsp. = _____ tbsp.

3. 1 pt. = _____ fluid oz. = _____ ml = _____ tbsp. = _____ tsp.

B. A child's amoxicillin dose is 20 mg/kg/day in divided doses every 8 hours.

1. This dose could also be written as 20 mg/_____ lb./day.

2. How many grams of amoxicillin would a 44-lb. child receive daily?

3. How many milligrams would this child receive per dose?

4. Amoxicillin is available as an oral suspension (125 mg/5 ml). How many teaspoonsful should this child receive per dose?

5. How many teaspoonsful should this child receive per day?

6. How many milliliters would you dispense for 10 days of therapy?

7. How many fluid ounces would you dispense for 10 days of therapy?

8. How many doses would the patient receive in 7 days?

C. How many milliliters of a liquid laxative should be dispensed if the dose prescribed is for 1 tbsp. q.i.d. for 3 days?

D. Flow rate calculations

1. If the flow rate for normal saline (NS) is 30 drops per minute over 6 hours, how many milliliters of NS would the patient receive (*assume 18 gtt./ml*)?

2. How many grams of NaCl would be administered (NS = 0.9 g of NaCl per 100 ml)?

E. A drug is administered by infusion at the rate of 1 mcg/lb./min. for anesthesia. If a 90-kg man is to receive a total of 0.85 mg of the drug:

    1. How long should the drug be infused?

    2. If the drug is available in a strength of 2 mg/5 ml, how many milliliters would the patient receive per minute?

    3. How many total milliliters would the patient receive?

F. How many milliliters of an injection containing 90 mg/ml of a drug should be administered to a 50-lb. child if the recommended dose is 6 mg per pound of body weight?

G. How many 125 mg antifungal tablets should be dispensed for a 100-lb. patient to provide a 30-day supply if the normal daily dose is 5 mg per pound of body weight?

H. An injectable antibiotic has a dose of 10 mg per kilogram of body weight. How many milliliters of a 125 mg/ml injection should be administered to a child weighing 66 lb.?

I. How many milliliters of digoxin injection 0.5 mg/2 ml would provide a 100 mcg dose?

J. A solution of sodium fluoride contains 1.1 mg/ml and has a dose of 15 drops. How many milligrams of sodium fluoride are in each dose if the dispensing dropper calibrates at 28 gtt./ml?

K. How many grams of diazepam will a patient receive in a week if he takes a 10 mg tablet t.i.d.?

L. 1. How many teaspoonful doses can a patient receive from a 6 fluid oz. bottle of cough syrup?

    2. For how long will this bottle of cough syrup last if the patient takes 1 dose every 4 hours?

M. How many milliliters of digoxin elixir 50 mcg/ml would provide a 0.25 mg dose?

N. 1. A patient is to receive ampicillin 250 mg q.i.d. for 10 days. How many capsules should be dispensed?

   2. If this prescription costs $16.80, how much does a dose count?

O. 1. How many milliliters of amoxicillin 250 mg/5 ml should be dispensed if the directions are to take 1 tsp. t.i.d. for 10 days?

   2. How many days will this dispensed volume last if the physician changes the directions to read: Take 1 1/2 tsp. b.i.d.?

P. 1. If the dose of a medication for an infant is 3 mg/lb., how much would a 12-lb. baby receive?

   2. How much of a drug available in an 8 mg/ml strength would provide the appropriate dose for this baby?

Q. 1. How many tablespoonful doses of potassium chloride can a patient receive from a 1 pt. bottle of potassium chloride?

   2. If the potassium chloride contains 10 g of potassium in every 100 ml, how many grams would a single dose contain?

   3. How many milligrams of potassium chloride would this 1 pt. bottle contain?

R. 1. A patient is to receive a liter of NS over 8 hours. How many milliliters will the patient receive each hour?

   2. How many drops per minute would this patient receive if the IV set delivers 10 gtt./ml?

S. 1. What is the body surface area of a 65-year-old patient who is 67 inches tall and weighs 152 lb.?

   2. If the recommended dose of a chemotherapy drug for this patient is 400 mcg/m^2, what would the dose be in milligrams?

Answers appear on pages 148–149.

Nomogram for Adults

Determination of body surface from height and mass[1]

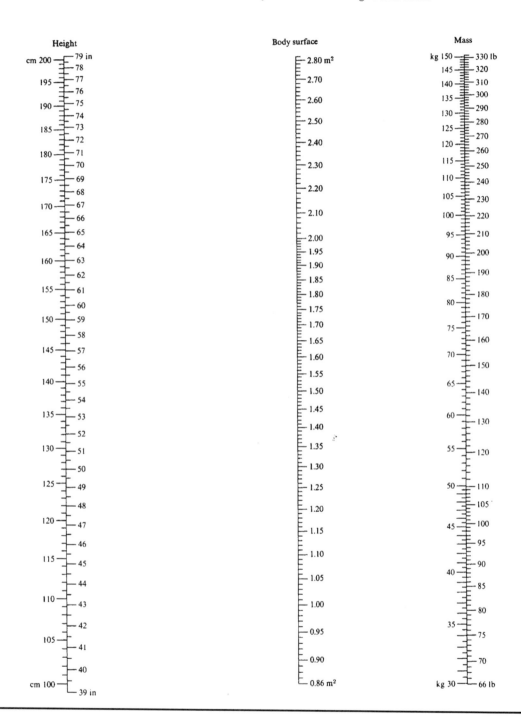

Height	Body surface	Mass

[1] From the formula of Du Bois and Du Bois, *Arch Intern Med,* 17, 863 (1916): $S = M^{0.425} \times H^{0.725} \times 71.84$, or $\log S = \log M \times 0.425 + \log H \times 0.725 + 1.8564$ (S = body surface in cm^2, M = mass in kg, H = height in cm).

Source: C. Lentner, Ed., *Geigy Scientific Tables,* 8th ed, vol 1, Basel: Ciba-Geigy; 1981: 226–7.

Notes:

Chapter Thirteen

Concentrations

I. Reducing and Enlarging Formulas

A. Pharmacists and technicians often have to prepare larger and/or smaller quantities than a recipe might call for.

1. Example: Recipe on a box for eight medium-size pancakes

Pancake mix	1 cup
Water	1/2 cup
Milk	1/4 cup
Eggs	2
Vegetable oil	2 tsp.

a. How much milk would be needed to make 16 pancakes?

b. How many eggs are needed to make four pancakes?

These problems can be solved by creating a factor using the amount the recipe calls for as a denominator and the amount desired as the numerator. Multiply this factor times each component in the recipe to "reduce" or "enlarge" the formula. In the above examples, the calculation would be:

$$\frac{16 \text{ pancakes}}{8 \text{ pancakes}} = 2 \,(1/4 \text{ cup of milk}) = 1/2 \text{ cup of milk}$$

$$\frac{4 \text{ pancakes}}{8 \text{ pancakes}} = 1/2 \,(2 \text{ eggs}) = 1 \text{ egg}$$

These problems can also be solved by using the principles of ratio and proportion:

$$\frac{1/4 \text{ cup of milk}}{8 \text{ pancakes}} = \frac{x}{16 \text{ pancakes}} \quad x = 1/2 \text{ cup}$$

$$\frac{2 \text{ eggs}}{8 \text{ pancakes}} = \frac{x}{4 \text{ pancakes}} \quad x = 1 \text{ egg}$$

II. Concentrations and Dilutions

A. Concentration may be expressed as a percentage. There are three types of percentages:
1. Weight-in-weight (w/w) percentage preparations
   a. Weight-in-weight percentage is used when the final product is a solid (powder, ointment, etc.) and the component for which you are measuring the percentage is also a solid. Units in the numerator and denominator must be the same (lb./lb., gr./gr., etc.).

   (1) Example: 2 g of sulfur in 100 g of a final ointment would be 2 g/100 g = 0.02 = 2% w/w

2. Volume-in-volume (v/v) percentage preparations
   a. Volume-in-volume percentage is used when the final product is a liquid (solution) and the component for which you are measuring the percentage is also a liquid. Units in the numerator must be the same as in the denominator (ml/ml, pt./pt., etc.).

   (1) Example: 5 ml of a flavoring oil in 100 ml of mouthwash would be
       5 ml/100 ml = 0.05 = 5% v/v

3. Weight-in-volume (w/v) percentage preparations
   a. Weight-in-volume percentage is used when the final product is a liquid, as indicated by the (v) in the denominator (e.g., suspensions), and the component for which you are measuring the percentage is a solid, as indicated by the (w) in the numerator. The numerator is always in grams and the denominator is always in milliliters (this differs from w/w and v/v percentages, in which the units could vary but have to be the same in both the numerator and denominator).

   (1) Example: 17 g of drug K in 100 ml of a final solution would be
       17 g/100 ml = 0.17 or 17% w/v

B. Ratio strength preparations
1. Ratios are just another way of expressing a percent (remember that percent means parts per 100). A 5% w/w product is 5 parts per 100 parts, or 5:100. A 20% v/v solution is 20 parts per 100 parts, or 20:100 (this could mean 20 ml of drug in 100 ml of solution, or 20 L in 100 L, etc.). A 15% w/v solution means 15 g of drug in 100 ml of solution, or 15:100. Ratio strength calculations are performed like percentage calculations.
   a. Example: 5% w/v = 5 g in 100 ml = 1 g in 20 ml = 1:20

2. Ratios should always be reduced so that the number "1" is written to the left of the colon (e.g., 1:100, not 2:200, even though these ratios are equal).
   a. Example: 3:15 could also be written:

$$\frac{3}{15} = \frac{1}{x}$$

x = 5, so 3:15 = 1:5

C. Stock solutions
1. Stock solutions are concentrated solutions from which weaker strength solutions can be easily made.

D. Dilutions of stock preparations
1. A dilution is performed when you take a certain percentage solution and add a 0% diluent to decrease the percentage concentration.
   a. Example: How much water would you add to 100 ml of a 15% potassium chloride solution to get a 5% final product?
   This problem cannot be solved by simple ratio and proportion because you are looking for an inverse relationship (i.e., the more solvent we add, the *lower* the percentage).

     (1) Easy method:

     (old volume)(old %) = (new volume)(new percent), which is also expressed as: (O.V.)(O.%) = (N.V.)(N.%)

     Step 1:   (100 ml)(15%) = (x)(5%)

     Step 2: $\dfrac{(100 \text{ ml})(15\%)}{(5\%)} = x \quad x = 300 \text{ ml}$

     Note: 300 ml is the final and total dilution you have made by adding 100 ml of 15% KCl to a certain volume of water. It is not the amount of water added.

     Answer: 300 ml final solution – 100 ml of 15% = 200 ml of H_2O added.

III. Alligation Methods

A. Alligation alternate method
1. Basic principles
   a. This technique is used for making dilutions when the diluent is zero percent or higher. Previous dilution examples used a zero percent diluent only.

   b. You can dilute to only an intermediate percent (i.e., you cannot add 10% to 20% and get a percent higher than 20% or lower than 10%). The final product will be somewhere between 10% and 20%.

2. Examples
   a. If you need a 10% sulfur ointment and have only 5% and 20% ointments available, use the alligation alternate method to determine how many "parts" of each will be needed to get the 10% final product. "Parts" can have any value (ml, gr., pinches, etc.) and all the parts, when added together, will equal the total parts of the final product, in this case the 10% ointment. Subtract 5% from 10% to get 5 parts. Subtract 10% from 20% to get 10 parts. The ratio is 5 parts of 20%:10 parts of 5%.

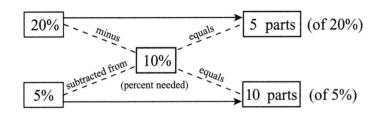

b. Using data from the previous example, prepare 1 kg of the 10% sulfur ointment.

Step 1: Add the parts, i.e., 5 + 10 = 15 parts (*Note:* The 15 parts represent the total quantities of the 20% and 5% ointments that are being combined. The "new" product, which is a 10% ointment, is equal to 15 parts.)

Step 2: 15 parts/1000 g = 10 parts/x
x = 667 g (of 5% ointment)

Step 3: 15 parts/1000 g = 5 parts/x
x = 333 g (of 20% ointment)

Note: Step 3 can be skipped by simply subtracting 667 from 1000.

Note: To compound 1000 g of 10%, add 667 g of 5% ointment to 333 g of 20% ointment.

B. Alligation medial method
   1. This method is used to obtain the average strength of a mixture of two or more substances whose concentration and percent strength are already known. This can also be used to check an alligation alternate problem.

   a. Example from the mixture in A.2. above:

   Step 1:   5 parts × 20% = 100 parts %
             10 parts × 5% = 50 parts %
             _____
             15 parts   150 parts %

   Step 2: $\dfrac{150 \text{ parts } \%}{15 \text{ parts } \%} = 10\%$

IV. Milliequivalents

A. Key terms and concepts
   1. Electrolytes
      a. Electrolytes are important for many bodily functions that require electrical activity such as nerve conduction and muscle contraction. Electrolyte replacement is usually ordered in units of milligrams or milliequivalents.

2. Milliequivalents
   a. A milliequivalent (mEq) is equal to the millimoles of H^+ or OH^- that will react with 1 mmol of an ion or compound. When an atom has the valence of "one," a milliequivalent (mEq) is simply equal to the atomic weight (AW) of the atom (e.g., $Na^+ = 23$, so there are 23 mg/mEq). A molecule like sodium chloride (NaCl) has a molecular weight (MW) of 58.5. Therefore, 1 mEq = 58.5 mg, and when the molecule dissociates, it yields 1 mEq Na^+ and 1 mEq Cl^-.

B. Converting to milliequivalents
   1. Example: If a solution contains 10 g of potassium chloride (KCl), how many mEq of K^+ does it contain? The AW of $K^+ = 39$ and the AW of $Cl^- = 35.5$. Therefore, the MW of KCl = 74.5.

      74.5 mg = 1 mEq
      10 g = 10,000 mg
      74.5 mg/1 mEq = 10,000 mg/x = 134 mEq

C. Divalent and trivalent ions
   1. Sometimes you will have an exception to the rule when you have divalent ions (e.g., Mg^{++}, Ca^{++}) and trivalent ions (e.g., Al^{+++}). In most cases when magnesium or calcium is involved in the molecule, 1 mEq is equal to 1/2 the MW. With aluminum-containing products, 1 mEq is equal to 1/3 the MW.

      a. Example: Calcium chloride ($CaCl_2$)   AW of $Ca^{++} = 40$ AW of $Cl^- = 35.5$
                    $40 + 35.5 + 35.5 = 111$ mg total weight
                    1 mEq = 111/2 (i.e., valence) = 55.5 mg

V. Dry Powders for Reconstitution

A. Many unstable medications are packaged as dry powders and must be dissolved in a solvent prior to dispensing. The most frequently encountered drugs requiring reconstitution are the antibiotics. In most cases, reconstitutions can be accomplished in three steps:
   1. Establish how much drug is in the vial or bottle.

   2. Calculate the powder volume displacement.

   3. Solve the problem using ratio and proportion.
      a. Example 1:   The label on a vial reads, "Add 9.2 ml of diluent to the vial to get 10 ml of a 100 mg/ml solution for injection." How many milliliters of the reconstituted solution would provide a 250 mg dose?

         (1) Step 1: $\dfrac{100\ mg}{1\ ml} = \dfrac{x}{10\ ml}$

                        x = 1000 mg per vial

         (2) Step 2:   not required at this point

(3) Step 3:

$$\frac{1000 \text{ mg}}{10 \text{ ml}} = \frac{250 \text{ mg}}{x}$$

$$x = 2.5 \text{ ml}$$

Note: This problem can also be solved by using the per-milliliter concentration of 100 mg/ml:

$$\frac{100 \text{ ml}}{1 \text{ ml}} = \frac{250 \text{ mg}}{x}$$

b. How much of the diluted solution for injection in Example 1 would you measure to get the 250 mg dose if you accidentally reconstituted with 11 ml of diluent?

   (1) Step 1: 1000 mg per vial

   (2) Step 2: If 9.2 ml of diluent, when mixed with the powder, yields 10 ml, then the powder volume displacement is 0.8 ml, i.e., $10 - 9.2 = 0.8$.

   (3) Step 3: 0.8 ml of powder + 11 ml of diluent = 11.8 ml

$$\frac{1000 \text{ mg}}{11.8 \text{ ml}} = \frac{250 \text{ mg}}{x}$$

$$x = 2.95 \text{ ml}$$

c. Example 2: You have been directed to reconstitute a 5 million unit vial of Drug A to a concentration of 500,000 units/ml. The drug has a powder volume displacement of 0.002 L. How many milliliters of diluent will you need to add to this vial?

   (1) Step 1: 5,000,000 units per vial

   (2) Step 2: 2 ml (given as 0.002 L)

   (3) Step 3: If you want 500,000 units per 1 ml, then

$$\frac{500,000 \text{ units}}{1 \text{ ml}} = \frac{5,000,000 \text{ units}}{x}$$

x = 10 ml (this is the total volume of the vial)
10 ml total volume − 2 ml powder
volume displacement = 8 ml of diluent to be added

VI. Sample Questions

A. Answer questions 1–3 using the following recipe for benzyl benzoate lotion:

Benzyl benzoate	250 ml
Triethanolamine	5 g
Oleic acid	20 g
Purified water to make	1000 ml

1. How many grams of triethanolamine are required to make 1 gal. of benzyl benzoate lotion? How many milligrams?

2. How many grains of oleic acid are required to make 1 pt. of benzyl benzoate lotion?

3. How many teaspoonsful of benzyl benzoate are there in 100 ml of the lotion?

B. 1. What percentage of sulfur would be in a product that contains 2 g of sulfur in 120 g of ointment?

2. How many milligrams of sulfur would be contained in 1 g of ointment?

C. What percentage of sulfur would be in a product containing 20 g of sulfur in 1 lb. of ointment?

D. 1. What percentage sulfur ointment would result from *adding* 50 g of sulfur to 120 g of petrolatum?

2. What is the percentage of petrolatum in the ointment?

E. Ninety grams of 25% zinc oxide ointment would contain how many grams of zinc oxide?

F. 1. What percentage of flavoring oil would be in a mouthwash that has 2 tbsp. of oil in 1 pt. of mouthwash?

2. How many milliliters of oil would be in 60 ml of the mouthwash?

G. Calculate the percentage of a preparation containing 7 g of drug K in 5 fluid oz. of a final product.

H. 1. Calculate the percentage of a preparation containing 1 lb. of drug K in 1 gal. of final product.

   2. What is the ratio strength of the final product?

I. 1. One pint of a 10% w/v suspension would contain _____ g of drug.

   2. One teaspoonful of this suspension would be what percent w/v?

J. One quart of a 1:50 w/v solution would be _____% and contain _____ g of active ingredient.

K. 1. How many milligrams per milliliter would be in a 6% w/v solution?

   2. What is the ratio strength of this solution?

L. A solution containing 2000 mg of a drug in 8 fluid oz. would be a _____ % w/v solution or a _____ ratio strength solution and contain _____ mg/ml.

M. 1. Convert 6:720 into a correctly written ratio strength.

   2. Express this value as a percentage strength.

N. 1. What is the resulting percentage of benzalkonium chloride obtained from diluting 1 fluid oz. of 17% benzalkonium chloride to 1 pt.?

   2. What is the final ratio strength?

   3. How many milligrams per milliliter are in the final dilution?

   4. How many grams per teaspoonful are in the initial 17% solution?

5. What is the percentage strength of 1 tsp. of the 17% solution *added* to 1 tbsp. of water?

6. How many grains of benzalkonium chloride are in 1 fluid oz. of 17% benzalkonium chloride?

7. How many grains of benzalkonium chloride are in the final 1 pt. dilution?

8. If 100 ml of a 1:200 drug solution is diluted to 1 L, what is the final ratio strength?

9. How many milligrams per teaspoonful doses are in the final dilution in question N.8?

O. 1. Can you mix a 20% ointment with a 5% ointment to make a 10% ointment?

2. If yes, how many grams of each component would be required to make 1 lb. of a 10% ointment?

3. If yes, how many grams of 10% ointment could be made if you had only 30 g of 20% and plenty of 5%?

P. 1. Can you mix a 20% ointment with a 15% ointment to make a 10% ointment?

2. If yes, how many grams of each component would be required to make 1 lb. of a 10% ointment?

3. If yes, how many grams of 10% ointment could be made if you had only 1 oz. of 20% and plenty of 15%?

Q. A liter of NS (0.9% sodium chloride) would contain _____ g of sodium chloride and _____ mEq of sodium? (AW of Na^+ = 23; AW of Cl^- = 35.5)

R. 1. If 100 ml of a solution contains 10 mEq of KCl, what is the percentage strength of potassium chloride? (MW of KCl = 74.5)

2. How many milligrams of KCl are required to prepare 1 L of this solution?

S. How many milliequivalents of calcium are in a tablespoonful of a solution containing 250 mg of calcium chloride ($CaCl_2$)? (AW of $Ca^{++} = 40$; $Cl^- = 35.5$)

T. What is the percentage strength of calcium chloride in the solution in the previous question?

U. How many milliequivalents of aluminum are in 1 g of aluminum hydroxide $Al (OH)_3$? (AW of $Al = 27$; $O = 16$; $H = 1$)

V. Answer questions V. 1–3 using the following prescription for ampicillin suspension:

Rx	Ampicillin 250 mg/5 ml
	Sig.: 1 tsp. q.i.d. × 10 d

1. How many milliliters would you dispense?

2. Assume that the instructions on the bottle of dry ampicillin powder for reconstitution require the addition of 160 ml of water to obtain the volume needed to correctly fill the prescription. What volume will the drug powder account for?

3. How many grams of ampicillin will the patient receive in 1 week?

W. The prescription below is a formula for 1 capsule to be extemporaneously compounded. How many 30 mg codeine sulfate tablets would be required to make 50 of these capsules?

Rx	Acetylsalicylic acid	325 mg
	Codeine sulfate	5 mg
	Sig.:	1 capsule q.4h p.r.n. pain

X. 1. How many 250 mg erythromycin tablets would be required to compound the prescription below?

Rx	E-Mycin 2%
	Alcohol q.s. 150 ml

2. What is the ratio strength of 1 tsp. of this prescription?

3. How many milligrams are in each milliliter of this prescription?

Y. The instructions on a vial for reconstitution state, "Add 12.8 ml of diluent to make 15 ml of a 500 mg/ml solution." You have on hand only 10 ml of the diluent, which you use for reconstitution.

1. How much drug is in the vial?

2. Does the total amount of drug in the vial change according to the amount of diluent added?

3. Does the amount of drug per milliliter vary with the amount of diluent added?

4. What is the powder volume displacement of the drug?

5. How many milliliters of the reconstituted solution, according to instructions on the vial, would provide a 2 g dose of the drug?

6. How many milliliters of the reconstituted solution made with 10 ml of diluent would provide a 2 g dose of the drug?

Z. 1. What is the percent strength of coal tar in a mixture of 1/2 kg of 3% coal tar ointment and 1500 g of 10% coal tar ointment?

2. What is the ratio strength of the coal tar mixture?

3. How many grams of coal tar are in 1 lb. of this mixture?

4. Can a 1:50 coal tar ointment be prepared by mixing the 3% and 10% coal tar ointments?

5. How many grams of coal tar should be added to the coal tar mixture to obtain an ointment containing 18% coal tar?

Answers appear on pages 149–152.

Notes:

Chapter Fourteen

Commercial Calculations

I. Determining Charges for Prescriptions and Medication Orders

A. Cost
1. Cost is the total paid for an item or items received as noted on an invoice.
   a. Example: The invoice states that you purchased 1/2 dozen mugs at $1.50 each, for a total of $9.00.

$$6 \times \$1.50 \text{ each} = \$9 \quad \text{or} \quad \frac{1 \text{ mug}}{\$1.50} \quad \frac{6 \text{ mugs}}{x}$$

B. Selling price
1. The selling price is 100% of the amount you will receive for the sale of an item (this includes your cost plus whatever amount you want as a profit).

C. Markup
1. Markup may be defined as the difference between your cost for a product and its actual selling price.

   Selling price = Cost + Markup

2. Example: For 30 tablets costing $0.40 each for which you want to receive $0.10 profit per tablet:

   Selling price = (30 × $0.40) + (30 × $0.10) = $15.00   or $12.00 + $3.00 = $15.00

D. Percent markup
1. The percent markup must be qualified before it can be defined. It must be stated as "percent markup on the selling price" or as "percent markup on the cost" to determine its true meaning. In retail practice, "percent markup" usually means percent of sales, not of cost.
   a. From the previous example, percent markup based on cost would be:

$$\frac{\text{Markup}}{\text{Cost}} = \frac{\$3.00}{\$12.00} = 0.25 = 25\%$$

E. Percent gross profit
    1. This is the percent based on the selling price instead of the cost.
        a. Example:

$$\text{Percent Gross Profit} = \frac{\text{Markup}}{\text{Selling Price}} = \frac{\$3.00}{\$15.00} = 0.20 = 20\%$$

F. Overhead
    1. It is important to consider overhead to determine the true profit of a business. Overhead includes operating costs such as utilities, taxes, insurance, and technician salaries.

G. Net profit
    1. Net profit can be defined as:
        a. Selling Price – (Cost of Goods + Overhead)

H. Inventory
    1. The inventory includes all items on hand and their cost.

I. Turnover
    1. Turnover refers to the number of times that merchandise is sold in a given length of time, normally 1 year.

II. Sample Questions

A. If you paid $0.20 per capsule for a bottle containing 100 capsules:

    1. What was the total cost of the bottle of capsules?

    2. If you wanted to make a $0.05 profit per capsule, what would be the selling price of 1 capsule?

    3. What would be the selling price of 30 capsules?

B. If a drug costs $50 and the selling price is $60:

    1. What is the markup?

    2. What is the percent markup based on cost?

3. What is the percent gross profit?

C. A patient bought a humidifier for $65 that was initially purchased by the pharmacy from a medical supply company for $45.

　1. What is the markup on the humidifier?

　2. What is the percent markup on the humidifier based on selling price?

　3. What is the percent markup on the humidifier based on cost?

　4. What would be the selling price if the supplier's price was the same, but the pharmacy owner charged a 72% markup based on cost?

D. The markup on 40 antibiotic capsules is $10, and a patient pays $65 for the entire prescription.

　1. What is the acquisition cost of the capsules for the pharmacy?

　2. What is the average cost per capsule for the patient?

　3. What is the markup on each capsule?

　4. If the patient takes 1 capsule b.i.d., what will be the cost to the patient for a week of therapy?

　5. What is the percent markup on the prescription based on cost?

　6. What is the percent markup on the prescription based on selling price?

Answers appear on page 152.

Notes:

Chapter Fifteen

Practice Questions

1. Which of the following products is not commercially available?

   a. Allopurinol 100 mg tablets
   b. Prednisone 5 mg tablets
   c. Alprazolam 5 mg tablets
   d. Indinavir sulfate 200 mg capsules

2. How many milligrams of zephiran chloride are needed to prepare 3 L of 1:30,000 solution?

   a. 0.1
   b. 1
   c. 10
   d. 100

3. How many grams of bacitracin (500 units/g) should be used to prepare 1 kg of bacitracin ointment containing 250 units of bacitracin per gram?

   a. 100
   b. 500
   c. 1000
   d. 250,000

4. Patient profiles should be created for:

   a. Patients who have chronic diseases (e.g., diabetes, hypertension)
   b. Patients who have prescriptions filled at the pharmacy regularly
   c. Every patient who presents a prescription to the pharmacy
   d. Any patient who has had 3 or more prescriptions filled at the pharmacy within a 6-month period

5. How many milliliters of a drug would be needed to provide a 10,000 mcg dose from a vial containing 0.1 g/10 ml?

   a. 1
   b. 10
   c. 100
   d. 1000

6. How many milligrams of ephedrine sulfate should be used to prepare the following prescription?

Rx	Sol. Ephedrine sulfate 1/4 % 30 ml
	Sig.: Use as directed

   a. 0.075
   b. 0.75
   c. 7.5
   d. 75

7. What is the generic name for Keflex®?

   a. Cefadroxil
   b. Cefixime
   c. Cephalexin
   d. Ceftazidime

8. An order is received to administer 5 mEq of potassium acetate per hour. The bag of intravenous fluid contains 30 mEq/L. How many drops per minute would be needed to provide the prescribed dose using a set that delivers 15 gtt./ml?

   a. 3
   b. 12
   c. 42
   d. 167

9. How many liters of a 0.9% aqueous sodium chloride solution can be made from 60 g of NaCl?

   a. 6.67
   b. 66.7
   c. 667
   d. 6667

10. How many grams of a 5% sulfur ointment must be mixed with 180 g of 20% sulfur ointment to prepare an 8% sulfur ointment?

   a. 45
   b. 90
   c. 180
   d. 720

11. If 5 ml of diluent are added to a vial containing 2 g of a drug for injection resulting in a final volume of 5.8 ml, what is the concentration in milligrams per milliliter of the drug in the reconstituted solution?

   a. 0.3
   b. 345
   c. 400
   d. 2035

12. Which prescription instructions would require 17 tablets to be dispensed?

    a. One tab. p.o. b.i.d. × 7 d
    b. One tab. a.c. & h.s. × 4 d
    c. One tab. t.i.d. × 3 d; 1 tab. b.i.d. × 3 d; 1 tab. q.d. × 3 d
    d. Two tab. b.i.d. × 2 d; 2 tab. q.d. × 3 d; 1 tab. q.d. × 3 d

13. Which of the following is not considered a dosage form?

    a. Powder
    b. Inhalation
    c. Paste
    d. Lotion

14. How many milliliters per hour would be required to infuse a dopamine dose of 5 mcg/kg/min. to a patient weighing 220 lb. if the dopamine is provided by a bag containing 800 mg/500 ml?

    a. 18.75
    b. 30.35
    c. 100.45
    d. 528.34

15. A physician prescribes 10 mg of a drug per kilogram of body weight once daily for 21 days for a patient weighing 264 lb. How many 200 mg tablets of the drug are required daily?

    a. 2
    b. 4
    c. 6
    d. 12

16. How many grams of potassium permanganate are required to prepare 2 qt. of 1:750 solution of potassium permanganate?

    a. 0.05
    b. 0.13
    c. 1.28
    d. 13

17. When the physician's instructions indicate that a drug should be taken sublingually, what directions might be included on the prescription label?

    a. Change the patch every 12 hours.
    b. Chew the medication thoroughly.
    c. Place the medication under the tongue until it dissolves.
    d. Use 0.5 ml in 2 ml of normal saline every 4 hours as needed.

18. The formula for zinc gelatin is:

Glycerin	400 g
Gelatin	150 g
Zinc oxide	100 g
Purified water	350 g

How much glycerin would be required to prepare 1 lb. of zinc gelatin?

    a. 182 g
    b. 192 g
    c. 519 g
    d. 1000 g

19. Which drug is used to treat patients with diabetes?

    a. Micronase
    b. Glucotrol
    c. Actos
    d. All of the above are used to treat diabetes.

20. How many 1/2 pt. bottles can be filled from a 2 gal. container of 10% potassium chloride?

    a. 16
    b. 32
    c. 64
    d. 128

21. A complete patient profile should include all of the following except:

    a. Nonprescription medications the patient is currently using
    b. Patient's annual income for reimbursement/payment information
    c. The brand name or manufacturer of the drug dispensed to fill the prescription
    d. Physical limitations and sociological factors specific to the patient

22. What is the percent alcohol contained in a mixture of 90 ml of elixir phenobarbital (14% alcohol), 100 ml of water, and 40 ml of high alcoholic elixir (78% alcohol)?

    a. 8%
    b. 19%
    c. 26%
    d. 64%

23. The technician must notify the pharmacist before modifying the patient profile in all cases except:

    a. The patient has experienced a stroke and has been prescribed a different antihypertensive medication.
    b. The strength or dosage of insulin differs from the patient's previous prescription.
    c. The patient is now covered by a new medical/prescription insurance company.
    d. The patient has become pregnant since the last prescription was filled.

24. If the dose of a drug is 35 mg/kg/day in 6 divided doses, how much would be given in each dose to a 38-lb. child?

    a. 17.3 mg
    b. 60.4 mg
    c. 101 mg
    d. 604 mg

25. How many micrograms of digoxin would be contained in 0.75 ml of an ampule labeled 0.5 mg/2 ml?

    a. 0.188
    b. 3.6
    c. 13.2
    d. 187.5

26. Patient information to be entered into the patient profile must include all of the following except:

    a. The pharmacist's signature confirming each item of information listed
    b. Patient's prescription history
    c. Patient allergies
    d. Reimbursement information

27. How many grams of potassium chloride are used in making 1 L of a solution containing 3 mEq of potassium per teaspoonful? (MW of KCl = 74.5)

    a. 44.7
    b. 74.5
    c. 223.5
    d. 44,700

28. How many milliliters of 20% merthiolate solution should be diluted with water to make 600 ml of a 0.5% merthiolate solution?

    a. 15
    b. 178
    c. 580
    d. 24,000

29. Using proper aseptic technique requires that all intravenous solutions must be:

    a. Filtered prior to dispensing
    b. Prepared in a laminar flow hood
    c. Administered in at least 50 ml of normal saline
    d. Refrigerated immediately after compounding

30. How many grams of yellow mercuric oxide must be *added* to 30 g of 1% yellow mercuric oxide ointment to prepare a 5% ointment?

    a. 0.8
    b. 1.26
    c. 28.9
    d. 713

31. An elixir is to contain 500 mcg of an alkaloid in each tablespoonful dose. How many milligrams of alkaloid would be required to prepare a liter of the elixir?

    a. 3.33
    b. 7.5
    c. 33.3
    d. 33,333

32. A prescription calls for 500 mg of tetracaine hydrochloride. If tetracaine hydrochloride costs $24.50 per 3 g, what is the cost of the quantity necessary to prepare the prescription?

    a. $1.25
    b. $2.85
    c. $4.08
    d. $147.72

33. How many milliliters of ampicillin 250 mg/5 ml should be dispensed to fill a prescription for 500 mg q.i.d. times 10 days?

    a. 100
    b. 150
    c. 200
    d. 400

34. An example of injectable drug cross-contamination that could cause a potentially fatal reaction would be:

    a. Cefamandole-cefazolin
    b. Gentamicin-amikacin
    c. Ampicillin-aminophylline
    d. Meperidine-codeine

35. All prescription labels must include:

    a. Trade name of the medication
    b. Generic name of the medication
    c. Address of the patient
    d. Expiration date

36. How many milliliters of 95% alcohol should be mixed with 30% alcohol to make 2000 ml of a 40% alcohol solution?

   a. 31
   b. 108
   c. 222
   d. 308

37. How many grams of benzethonium chloride should be used in preparing 4 pt. of a 1:1000 solution of benzethonium chloride?

   a. 1.92
   b. 3.86
   c. 20
   d. 38

38. How many milliequivalents of potassium gluconate are there in 2 tbsp. of a 30% potassium gluconate solution? (MW potassium gluconate = 234; valence = 1)
   a. 21.65
   b. 38.46
   c. 390
   d. 9000

39. The dose of a drug for a 150-lb. patient is 280 mg. How many milliliters of a product containing 180 mg/tsp. would provide the appropriate dose?

   a. 4.9
   b. 7.8
   c. 12.7
   d. 18.2

40. By law, patient package inserts *must* be provided to all patients receiving:

   a. A prescription medication for the first time only
   b. Certain prescription medications for the first time only
   c. Prescription medications in all instances, including refills
   d. Certain medications in all instances, including refills

41. The principle behind the use of the horizontal laminar airflow hood is:

   a. Air from the sterile compounding room is pumped directly through the hood horizontally to minimize contamination from microorganisms.
   b. Filtered air flows from the hood toward the operator to provide a relatively clean work area.
   c. Filtered air is provided in straight, parallel lines, flowing downward.
   d. The operator is protected from the possible hazardous effects of cytotoxic agents.

42. How many milliliters of a 0.5% sodium sulfate solution should be mixed with a 5% sodium sulfate solution to make a liter of 2% solution?

    a. 250
    b. 333
    c. 500
    d. 667

43. There are 18 g of an expectorant in a liter of a cough syrup. How many grains of expectorant are contained in a teaspoonful dose of the cough syrup?

    a. 0.09
    b. 1.38
    c. 5.84
    d. 90

44. How many capsules, each containing 1 3/8 gr. of a drug, can be filled completely from a 28 g bottle of the drug?

    a. 24
    b. 32
    c. 313
    d. 431

45. If 4 fluid oz. of a solution cost $8.75, how much would a tablespoonful cost?

    a. $0.36
    b. $1.09
    c. $4.38
    d. $6.25

46. How many milliequivalents of potassium are in 2 g of potassium penicillin V if the molecular weight is 389 and the valence is 1?

    a. 5.14
    b. 78.2
    c. 154.6
    d. 389.3

47. What would be the infusion rate for a 50 mg/ml magnesium sulfate solution to provide 1.2 g/hr.?

    a. 0.4 ml/min.
    b. 2.5 ml/min.
    c. 20 ml/min.
    d. 24 ml/min.

48. A neonate in the nursery weighing 5 lb. 8 oz. requires 2.5 mg/kg of gentamicin. How many milliliters of solution containing 20 mg/ml should be administered?

    a. 0.029
    b. 0.31
    c. 2.5
    d. 6.3

49. A solution contains 5 mEq of calcium per 50 ml. How many milligrams of calcium would be contained in a liter of this solution? (AW calcium = 40; valence = 2)

    a. 20
    b. 100
    c. 2000
    d. 4000

50. How many milligrams of benzocaine are needed to prepare the following prescription?

Rx	Glycerin		2.5%
	Benzocaine		2%
	Hydrophilic ung.	q.s.	60 g

    a. 1.2
    b. 12
    c. 120
    d. 1200

51. How many grains of ephedrine are left in a 437.5 gr. bottle of ephedrine after compounding 400 capsules each containing 3/8 gr. of ephedrine?

    a. 28.5
    b. 73.2
    c. 150.8
    d. 287.5

52. Which of the following is not a reliable factor to consider when identifying a manufacturing source for a particular drug?

    a. Purchase price
    b. Quantity of medication used by the pharmacy each year
    c. Policies that are used by other pharmacies for ordering their drug inventories
    d. Delivery turn-around time for orders

53. The instructions on a nafcillin vial say to add 3.4 ml of sterile water to the 1 g vial resulting in 4.1 ml of solution. How many milliliters would provide a 675 mg dose?

    a. 0.36
    b. 1.92
    c. 2.31
    d. 2.77

54. Assume in the previous question that you accidentally used 4.3 ml of sterile water to reconstitute the 1 g vial of nafcillin. How many milliliters of this new solution would provide the 675 mg dose?

    a. 0.7
    b. 2.8
    c. 3.4
    d. 4.3

55. How many milliliters of a 0.1% solution can be made from 75 mg of a chemical?

    a. 10 ml
    b. 75 ml
    c. 100 ml
    d. 750 ml

56. A compounded ointment requires it to be heated to 65°C. What would this reading be on a Fahrenheit thermometer?

    a. 18
    b. 68
    c. 149
    d. 172

57. Upon receipt, all of the following products should be stored under refrigeration except:

    a. Insulin
    b. Chlorpromazine concentrate
    c. Mycostatin® pastilles
    d. Famotidine injection

58. One gram of dextrose provides 3.4 calories. How many calories would be provided by a liter of a 50% dextrose solution?

    a. 1.7
    b. 17
    c. 170
    d. 1700

59. How many grams of coal tar are needed to compound 1 lb. of this prescription?

Rx	Coal tar		2 g
	Zinc oxide paste	q.s.	60 g

   a. 2.3
   b. 15.1
   c. 16.2
   d. 21.6

60. An intravenous solution containing 20,000 units of heparin in 500 ml of 0.45% sodium chloride solution is to be infused to provide 1000 units of heparin per hour. How many drops per minute should be infused to deliver the desired dose if the IV set calibrates at 15 gtt./ml?

   a. 0.42
   b. 6
   c. 16
   d. 32

61. How many colchicine tablets containing 600 mcg each can be prepared from 40 g of colchicine?

   a. 66
   b. 666
   c. 6666
   d. 66,666

62. How many grams of a 5% benzocaine ointment can be prepared by diluting 1 lb. of 20% benzocaine ointment with white petrolatum?

   a. 129
   b. 642
   c. 735
   d. 1816

63. How many milligrams of pilocarpine nitrate are required to prepare 15 ml of an ophthalmic solution containing 0.25% pilocarpine nitrate?

   a. 0.61
   b. 18.2
   c. 37.5
   d. 380.9

64. How many 2.25 g sodium chloride tablets would be required to prepare 5 L of a 0.9% solution of sodium chloride?

   a. 20
   b. 70
   c. 100
   d. 2000

65. From the following formula, determine how many grams of calcium carbonate would be required to prepare 1 kg of the powder:

Magnesium oxide	1 part
Calcium carbonate	6 parts
Sodium bicarbonate	8 parts

   a. 0.1
   b. 30
   c. 400
   d. 750

66. Prochlorperazine injection is available in 10 ml multiple dose vials containing 5 mg/ml. How many 2.5 mg doses can be withdrawn from a single vial?

   a. 4
   b. 5
   c. 20
   d. 40

67. How many milliliters of water should be *added* to a quart of 10% boric acid solution to make a 3% solution?

   a. 1120
   b. 1600
   c. 2240
   d. 3200

68. Which drug targets estrogen production to treat cancer?

   a. Cytarabine
   b. Methotrexate
   c. Arimidex
   d. Daunorubicin

69. Ten pounds of a drug are required to make 340,000 tablets. How many kilograms of drug are required to make 170,000 tablets?

   a. 2.27
   b. 22.7
   c. 227
   d. 2270

70. Which of the following statements is true regarding investigational drugs?

    a. Technicians may not handle or dispense investigational drugs.
    b. Investigational drugs may be dispensed on a particular schedule that may be unusual for other drugs.
    c. Investigational drugs are cytotoxic agents that require special precautions.
    d. Study coordinators are responsible for maintaining only dispensing records for investigational drugs.

71. If a drug contains 50 mg of an expectorant per tablespoon, how many grams would be in a quart of this medication?

    a. 3.2
    b. 9.6
    c. 3200
    d. 9600

72. If an alprazolam tablet contains 0.25 mg of active ingredient, how many grains would be in 50 tablets?

    a. 0.086
    b. 0.192
    c. 0.811
    d. 12.53

73. Restricted drugs:

    a. Are usually prescribed for patients who have failed other therapies
    b. Have not been approved by FDA
    c. Are mostly used in younger patients because of severe side effects
    d. Have a broad range of uses in many disease states

74. A 2 ml vial of tobramycin sulfate contains 80 mg of the drug. How many milliliters of the injection would be required to obtain 0.02 g of tobramycin sulfate?

    a. 0.25
    b. 0.5
    c. 2.5
    d. 5.0

75. An IV set delivers 18 drops for every milliliter. How many drops would be in a 0.5 L bag of intravenous solution?

    a. 300
    b. 600
    c. 9000
    d. 18,000

76. Tamoxifen is primarily used to treat:

    a. Osteosarcoma
    b. Breast neoplasms
    c. Lymphoma
    d. Estrogen deficiency

77. How many milligrams of doxorubicin would be administered in a single dose to a 20-kg 96-cm-tall, 6-year-old child with a body surface area of approximately 0.7 m^2 if the intravenous dose is 30 mg per square meter of body surface area daily on 3 successive days every 4 weeks?

    a. 21
    b. 30
    c. 64
    d. 356

78. A patient sends a prescription that reads:

Depakote ER	500 mg
Sig.:	1 tab. (500 mg) b.i.d.
Dispense:	90 days supply

    How many tablets would you dispense?

    a. 90
    b. 60
    c. 360
    d. 180

79. How many milliliters of an injection containing 0.5 mg/ml of a drug would provide a 250 mcg dose?

    a. 0.2
    b. 0.5
    c. 2
    d. 5

80. How many milligrams of phenytoin would a 46-lb. child receive if the physician wants the child to receive 4 mg of phenytoin per kilogram of body weight?

    a. 24
    b. 84
    c. 184
    d. 404

81. A patient presents a prescription that reads:

Metformin	500 mg
Sig.:	2 tab. b.i.d.
Dispense:	90 days supply

How many tablets would you dispense?

a. 240
b. 120
c. 180
d. 360

82. In preparing a pint of elixir containing 200 mcg of an alkaloid per tablespoonful, how many milligrams of the alkaloid would you need to use?

a. 6.4
b. 19.2
c. 6400
d. 19,200

83. The dose of gentamicin is 2.5 mg/kg administered every 12 hours. What would be the daily dose for an 8.8-lb. baby?

a. 10
b. 20
c. 48
d. 96

84. Lotronex® (alosetron) must never be dispensed to:

a. Women of childbearing age
b. Men less than 20 years of age
c. Patients with irritable bowel syndrome
d. Patients without a prescribing program sticker on a written prescription

85. An intravenous solution is ordered to provide a patient 1 L of D5W over 8 hours. How many milliliters per minute would the patient receive?

a. 2.08
b. 9.44
c. 16.62
d. 125

86. If diphenhydramine elixir contains 12.5 mg diphenhydramine per teaspoonful, how many grams would be required to prepare a quart of the elixir?

    a. 2.4
    b. 800
    c. 1200
    d. 2400

87. Clozapine (Clozaril®):

    a. May cause life-threatening side effects
    b. Is effective in treating severe, disfiguring nodular acne and certain other skin diseases when other therapies have failed
    c. Has been approved by the FDA and is commonly used today
    d. May be dispensed in quantities for a 3-month supply

Use the following information for questions 88–90:

Starch	250 g
Sucrose	150 g
Magnesium sulfate	0.75 g
Lactose	125 g
Yield:	1000 placebo tablets

88. How many kilograms of sucrose would be needed to prepare 50,000 placebo tablets?

    a. 7.5
    b. 12.5
    c. 7500
    d. 12,500

89. How many placebo tablets would contain 5 lb. of starch?

    a. 9.08
    b. 90.8
    c. 908
    d. 9080

90. What is the percent of magnesium sulfate in each tablet?

    a. 0.00143
    b. 0.0143
    c. 0.143
    d. 1.43

Use the following information for questions 91–95:

> The label on a vial directs you to "add 7.8 ml of sterile water" to prepare a 10 ml "multidose" vial of a 100 mg/ml injection.

91. What is the dry powder volume of the drug in this vial?

    a. 0.22
    b. 2.2
    c. 12.2
    d. Cannot be determined

92. How many milliliters of reconstituted solution for injection would provide a 300 mg dose?

    a. 0.2
    b. 0.3
    c. 3
    d. 20

93. How many grams of the drug are in the vial?

    a. 1
    b. 10
    c. 100
    d. 1000

94. If a patient is to receive 250 mg q.i.d. for10 days, how many multidose vials will be required?

    a. 1
    b. 10
    c. 100
    d. 1000

95. How many milliliters of the reconstituted solution would provide a 250 mg dose if the vial was accidentally reconstituted with 9.8 ml of sterile water?

    a. 0.3
    b. 3
    c. 30
    d. Cannot be done

Use the following information for questions 96–99:

> A physician orders a patient to receive 4 million units of ampicillin in a 1000 ml bag of an intravenous solution to be infused over 12 hours. The nurse has elected to use an IV set that delivers 15 gtt./ml.

96. How many milliliters of solution will the patient receive per hour?

    a. 0.83
    b. 8.3
    c. 83.3
    d. 830

97. How many units of ampicillin will the patient receive per minute?

    a. 5.55
    b. 55.5
    c. 555
    d. 5555

98. What is the flow rate in milliliters per minute?

    a. 1.39
    b. 13.9
    c. 139
    d. Cannot be determined

99. How many drops per hour will the patient receive?

    a. 1.25
    b. 12.5
    c. 125
    d. 1250

Use the following information for questions 100 and 101:

> Precipitated sulfur   5%
> Benzocaine   1:500
> Zinc oxide paste ad 120 g

100. How many milligrams of benzocaine are contained in this prescription?

    a. 0.24
    b. 2.4
    c. 24
    d. 240

101. How many grams of precipitated sulfur would be required to prepare 1 kg of this product?

    a. 0.5
    b. 5
    c. 50
    d. 500

102. Cytotoxic drugs:

    a. Have all been shown to have an antitestosterone component
    b. Are primarily used to treat breast cancer
    c. Do not pose a hazard to health care professionals when properly handled and dispensed
    d. Do not require special labeling

103. What is the percent strength of ichthammol in a mixture of 1 kg each of ichthammol ointments containing 10%, 15%, and 20%?

    a. 10
    b. 15
    c. 25
    d. 45

Use the following information for questions 104–106:

A fluid ounce of 20% boric acid solution is diluted to 1000 ml with water.

104. What is the percent strength of the dilution?

    a. 0.006
    b. 0.06
    c. 0.6
    d. 6

105. What is the ratio strength of the dilution?

    a. 1:2847
    b. 1:1776
    c. 1:345
    d. 1:167

106. How many milligrams of boric acid are in a tablespoonful of the final dilution?

    a. 0.03
    b. 0.09
    c. 30
    d. 90

107. Thalidomide:

    a. May be the most effective therapy for irritable bowel syndrome in women who have failed to respond to conventional therapy

    b. Does not require registration of the patient or physician

    c. Is an effective treatment for erythema nodosum leprosum

    d. May be dispensed for a 90-day supply

Use the following information for questions 108–111:

> A 95% alcohol solution is mixed with 45% alcohol solution to make a 55% solution.

108. In what proportions should the alcohols be mixed to prepare the 55% solution?

    a. 40 parts 95% and 10 parts 45%

    b. 30 parts 95% and 20 parts 45%

    c. 20 parts 95% and 30 parts 45%

    d. 10 parts 95% and 40 parts 45%

109. How many milliliters of the 95% alcohol solution are required to prepare a liter of the 55% solution?

    a. 100

    b. 200

    c. 400

    d. 800

110. How many milliliters of the 45% alcohol solution are required to prepare a liter of the 55% solution?

    a. 100

    b. 200

    c. 400

    d. 800

111. How many milliliters of the 55% mixture can be prepared by mixing 45% and 95% alcohol solutions if you have only a pint of 95% alcohol and 3 gal. of 45% alcohol?

    a. 1200

    b. 2400

    c. 4300

    d. 8800

112. Accutane®:

    a. Is commonly used to treat acne in patients from 16 to 45 years old

    b. Effectively treats disfiguring nodular acne

    c. Effectively treats actinic onchomycosis on a limited basis

    d. Causes a severe interaction when patient is also taking isotretinoin

Use the following information for questions 113–116:

> A pharmacist purchases a box containing a dozen tubes of zinc oxide for $14.88 and sells the tubes of ointment for $2.69 each.

113. What is the markup on each tube?
    a. $0.88
    b. $1.25
    c. $1.45
    d. $2.48

114. What is the percent markup based on selling price?
    a. 22%
    b. 48%
    c. 54%
    d. 117%

115. What is the percent markup based on cost?
    a. 22%
    b. 48%
    c. 54%
    d. 117%

116. What would a tube cost if the store offered a 30% discount on all topical products?
    a. $0.65
    b. $1.16
    c. $1.88
    d. $3.49

117. Which drug is commonly used to treat diabetes?
    a. Gabapentin
    b. Sular
    c. Metformin
    d. Sotalol

118. Amitriptyline is used to treat:
    a. High blood pressure
    b. Depression
    c. Diabetes
    d. None of the above

119. Simvastatin is the generic name for:
    a. Lipitor®
    b. Tricor®
    c. Advicor®
    d. Zocor®

120. Which one of these agents is not used specifically to treat cancer?
    a. Daunorubicin
    b. Cytarabine
    c. Propafenone
    d. Tamoxifen

121. Alendronate 35 mg:

    a. Is the generic name for Actonel® 35 mg
    b. Is available in a formulation with calcium
    c. Is taken once weekly
    d. All of the above

Use the following information for questions 122–126:

A liter bottle of an enteral feeding formulation contains the following:

1200 calories	1200 mg sodium
2000 mg potassium	43 g protein
170 g carbohydrates	10 g fiber
39 g fat	

122. How many calories would a patient receive from 1500 ml of this formulation?

    a. 600
    b. 1200
    c. 1800
    d. 2400

123. Approximately how many milligrams of protein would a patient receive in an hour if the administration rate is 60 ml/hr.?

    a. 2.6
    b. 26
    c. 260
    d. 2600

124. How many total kilograms of fat and carbohydrates would a patient receive from 2 bottles of this formulation?

    a. 0.418
    b. 4.18
    c. 41.8
    d. 418

125. What would be the administration rate in milliliters per hour of the formulation if a physician wants the patient to receive 160 mg potassium every hour?

    a. 8
    b. 40
    c. 60
    d. 80

126. How many micrograms of fiber would be in a tablespoonful of this formulation?

    a. 0.15
    b. 1.5
    c. 150
    d. 150,000

Answers appear on pages 152–158.

Notes:

Answer Key

Answer Key To Sample and Practice Questions

Chapter One

A.   4
B.   4
C.1.   true
C.2.   false

(If a patient requests a refill, the technician should notify the pharmacist.)

D.1.   yes
D.2.   yes
D.3.   no
D.4.   yes
D.5.   no
D.6.   no
D.7.   yes
D.8.   no
D.9.   yes
D.10.   yes
D.11.   no
D.12.   no
D.13.   yes
D.14.   no
D.15.   yes
D.16.   no
D.17.   yes
E.1.   Take two tablets by mouth 4 times a day.
E.2.   Take one capsule before meals and at bedtime.
E.3.   Inject 5 mg intramuscularly every 3–4 hours as needed for nausea.
E.4.   Instill 1 drop into right eye every 12 hours.
E.5.   Instill 2–3 drops into each ear 3 times a day.
E.6.   Instill 1 drop into each ear twice daily.

F.   3
G.   5

Chapter Two

A.1.   false
A.2.   true
A.3.   true
A.4.   false
B.   5

Chapter Three

A.1.   false
A.2.   true
A.3.   false
B.   2
C.   5
D.1.   c
D.2.   e
D.3.   l
D.4.   k
D.5.   i
D.6.   b
D.7.   a
D.8.   j
D.9.   g
D.10.   d
D.11.   f
D.12.   h
E.   5

Chapter Four

A.	2
B.1.	false
B.2.	false
C.	1
D.1.	c
D.2.	c
D.3.	a
D.4.	c
D.5.	a
D.6.	c
D.7.	a
D.8.	a
D.9.	c
D.10.	b

Chapter Five

A.	5
B.	4
C.	5
D.1.	false
D.2.	true
D.3.	false
D.4.	true
D.5.	false
E.	3
F.	4

Chapter Six

A.	5
B.	5
C.	5
D.1.	false
D.2.	false
D.3.	true
D.4.	false
D.5.	true
D.6	false
E.	5

Chapter Seven

A.	3
B.	5
C.1.	false
C.2.	false
C.3.	false
C.4.	true
C.5.	true
D.	4

Chapter Eight

A.	5
B.	1

Chapter Nine

A.1. $\dfrac{10 \div 5}{75 \div 5} = \dfrac{2}{15}$

A.2. $\dfrac{8 \div 8}{16 \div 8} = \dfrac{1}{2}$

A.3. $\dfrac{3 \div 3}{15 \div 3} = \dfrac{1}{5}$

A.4. 60/186 = 30/93 = 10/31

B.1. 5 = 5/1

B.2. 3 2/3 = 11/3

C.1. 30/64, 12/64, 7/64

C.2. 18/24, 21/24, 10/24

D. 15/4 = 3 3/4

E. 3/4 + 1 1/8 = 6/8 + 9/8 = 15/8 = 1 7/8

F. 7 5/8 − 1 1/3 = 61/8 − 4/3 = 183/24 − 32/24 = 151/24 = 6 7/24

G. 1 3/4 × 3 = 7/4 × 3/1 = 21/4 = 5 1/4

H. 1/2 ÷ 5 = 1/2 ÷ 5/1 = 1/2 × 1/5 = 1/10

I. 3/16 ÷ 1 1/2 = 3/16 ÷ 3/2 = 3/16 × 2/3 = 6/48 = 1/8

J.1. 0.07 = 7/100

J.2. 0.077 = 77/1000

J.3. 5.0125 = 5 125/10,000 = 5 1/80

K.1. 3/8 = 0.375

K.2.	2 7/13 = 33/13 = 2.54
L.1.	3.75 − 1/2 = 3.75 − 0.5 = 3.25
L.2.	3/4 × 2.5 = 0.75 × 2.5 = 1.875
L.3.	2 3/8 ÷ 0.5 = 2.375 ÷ 0.5 = 4.75
M.1.	29 = XXIX
M.2.	47 = XLVII
M.3.	86 = LXXXVI
M.4.	1154 = MCLIV
N.1.	LXXVIII = 78
N.2.	CXIII = 113
N.3.	XCIV = 94
N.4.	MCMLXI = 1961
O.	3/8 = 0.375
	0.375 ÷ 0.0125 = 30 doses

P. Step 1: $2 \times 1.25 = 2.5$
$3 \times 1.75 = 5.25$
_____
7.75 oz. dispensed
Step 2: $8 - 7.75 = 0.25$ oz. remaining in the bottle

Q.	1/200 ÷ 1/40 = 1/200 × 40/1 = 40/200 = 1/5 tablet
R.	1/150 ÷ 1/400 = 1/150 × 400/1 = 400/150 = 2 2/3
S.	10 × 44 = 440 = CDXL
T.	9 + 6 + 60 = 75 g
U.	515 − 66 = 449 lb.
V.	20 × 445 = 8900 mg
W.	251 × 4 = 1004 = MIV
X.	120 × 4 = 480 = CDLXXX
Y.1.	3/1 × 3/8 = 9/8 = 1 1/8 lb.
Y.2.	1 1/8 = 9/8 = 18/16
	18/16 − 3/16 = 15/16 lb.
Z.	1/150 × 4 = 4/150 = 0.0267 gr.
AA.1.	120 ml/24 tsp. = 5 ml/1 tsp.
AA.2.	24 tsp./0.75 tsp. = 32
BB.	24 × 325 = 7800 mg
CC.1.	100 × 9/8 = 900/8 = 112.5 g
CC.2.	200 − 112.5 = 87.5 g
DD.	1635/109 = 15
EE.	0.75/0.004 = 187.5 doses

Chapter Ten

A.1. 72% = 72/100 = 0.72
A.2. 0.35 = 35% = 35/100 = 7/20
A.3. 25% = 25/100 = 25:100
A.4. 0.182 = 18.2%
A.5. 3/8 = 0.375 = 37.5%

B.1. $40
A/B = C/D
10 lb./$200 = 2 lb./x
(x) (10 lb.) = ($200) (2 lb.)
$$x = \frac{(\$200) (2\ lb.)}{10\ lb.}$$
x = $40

B.2. 1.25 lb.
A/B = C/D
10 lb./$200 = x/$25
($25) (10 lb.) = ($200) (x)
$$(\$25) (10\ lb.) = \frac{x}{(\$200)}$$
x = 1.25 lb.

B.3. $12.50
Step 1: A/B = C/D
1 lb./16 oz. = 10 lb./x
$$(10\ lb.) (16\ oz.) = \frac{x}{1\ lb.}$$
x = 160 oz. (160 oz. cost $200 as mentioned earlier)
Step 2: A/B = C/D
160 oz./$200 = 10 oz./x
(10 oz.) ($200) = (160 oz.) (x)
$$(10\ oz.) (\$200) = \frac{x}{160\ oz.}$$
x = $12.50

C. 5.46 g
1000 tab./11.5 g = 475 tab./x
x = 5.46 g

D. 160 mg
5 mg/15 ml = x/480 ml
x = 160 mg

E. 32,500 mg
2 tab./650 mg = 100 tab./x
x = 32,500 mg

F. 300 tablets
7 tab./35 mg = x/1500 mg
x = 300 tablets

G. $52.20
$0.58/1 tab. = x/90 tab.
x = $52.20

H. 0.65 g
1 cap./0.0325 g = 20 cap./x
x = 0.65 g

I. $206.49
385 lb./$795 = 100 lb./x
x = $206.49

J. 78.64 kg
2.2 lb./1 kg = 173 lb./x
x = 78.64 kg

K. 300,000 units
6,000,000 units/10 ml = x/0.5 ml
x = 300,000 units

L. 300 ml
5 ml/1 min. = x/60 min.
x = 300 ml

M. 5250 mg
750 mg/1 day = x/7 days
x = 5250 mg

N. 11.2 mg
28 mg/3 ml = x/1.2 ml
x = 11.2 mg

O. 1.5 g
10 g/100 ml = x/15 ml
x = 1.5 g

P. $8.96
15 ml/$0.28 = 480 ml/x
x = $8.96

Q.1. $1.35
12 bottles/$1.80 = 9 bottles/x
x = $1.35

Q.2. $18.00
1 dozen/$1.80 = 10 dozen/x
x = $18.00

R.1. 4.5 min.
60 sec./1 min. = 270 sec./x
x = 4.5 min.

R.2. 100 Rx
7.5 hr. × 60 min./hr. = 450 min.
1 Rx/4.5 min. = x/450 min.
x = 100 Rx

S.1. 90 tablets
3 tab./day = x/30 days
x = 90 tablets

S.2. 450 mg
5 mg/1 tab. = x/90 tab.
x = 450 mg

T.1. 4.54/454 = 0.01

T.2. 0.01 = 1/100 = 1%

U. 20/100 = 2/10 = 1/5 = 1:5

V.1. $3.67
6 oz./$88 = 1/4/x
x = $3.67

V.2. 0.068 oz.
6 oz./$88 = x/$1
x = 0.068 oz.

W.1. 3/16 g
100/3/8 = 50/x
x = 3/16 g

W.2. 3/16 = 0.1875 = 18.75%

Chapter Eleven

A.1. 225 km = 225,000 m
1 km/1000 m = 225 km/x

A.2. 525 g = 0.525 kg
1 kg/1000 g = x/525 g

A.3. 5 g = 5000 mg
1 g/1000 mg = 5 g/x
5 g = 5,000,000 mcg
1 g/1,000,000 mcg = 5 g/x

A.4. 350 ml = 0.35 L
1 L/1000 ml = x/350 ml

B.1. 480 ml
30 ml/1 oz. = x/16 oz.

B.2. 32 fluid oz.
1 pt. /16 fluid oz.= 2 pt./x

B.3. 8 pints
2 pt./1 qt. = x/4 qt.
128 fluid ounces
16 oz./1 pt. = x/8 pt.

C.1. 7000 gr.
1 oz./437.5 gr.= 16 oz./x

C.2. 7.62 cm
1 inch/2.54 cm = 3 inches/x

D.1.   0.065 g
        1 g/15.4 gr. = x/1 gr.
        65 mg
        1 g/1000 mg = 0.065 g/x

D.2.   437.5 gr.
        28.4 g
        1 g/15.4 gr. = x/437.5 gr.

D.3.   16 oz.
        454 g
        1 oz./28.4 g = 16 oz./x
        7000 gr.
        1 g/15.4 gr. = 454 g/x
        0.454 kg
        1 kg/1000 g = x/454 g

D.4.   2.2 lb.
        454 g/1 lb. = 1000 g/x

E.1.   16 fluid oz.
        480 ml
        1 oz./30 ml = 16 oz./x

E.2.   128 fluid oz.
        16 oz./1 pt. = x/8 pt.
        3840 ml
        1 oz./30 ml = 128 oz./x
        3.84 L
        1 L/1000 ml = x/3840 ml

F.   68°F
        °F = 32 + 9/5 °C
        °F = 32 + 9/5 (20)
        °F = 32 + 36
        °F = 68 °

G.   100°C
        °C = 5/9 (°F – 32)
        °C = 5/9 (212 – 32)
        °C = 5/9 (180)
        °C = 100

H.   1538 tablets
        Step 1: 0.5 kg = 500 g = 500,000 mg
        Step 2: 325 mg/1 tab. = 500,000 mg/x
        x = 1538 tablets

I.   111.8 kg
        2.2 lb./1 kg = 246 lb./x
        x = 111.8 kg

J.   8000 mcg
        Step 1: 40 mg = 40,000 mcg
        Step 2: 40,000 mcg/10 ml = x/2 ml
        x = 8000 mcg

K.   38.5 gr.
        Step 1: 10 g/1000 ml = x/250 ml
        x = 2.5 g
        Step 2: 1 g/15.4 gr. = 2.5 g/x
        x = 38.5 gr.

L.1.   28.8 oz.
        16 oz./1 lb. = x/1.8 lb.
        x = 28.8 oz.

L.2. $252
        1 oz./$8.75 = 28.8 oz./x
        x = $252

L.3. $6.56
        1 oz./$8.75 = 3/4 oz./x
        x = $6.56

M.1.   96 bottles
        4 oz./1 bottle = 384 oz./x
        x = 96 bottles

M.2. $1.25
        128 oz./$40 = 4 oz./x
        x = $1.25

N.1.   800,000 × 15 = 12,000,000 mg =
        12,000 g = 12 kg

N.2.   26.43 lb.
        454 g/1 lb. = 12,000 g/x
        x = 26.43 lb.

N.3.   423 oz.
        1 lb./16 oz. = 26.43 lb./x
        x = 423 oz.

N.4. $6281
        1 oz./$14.85 = 423 oz./x
        x = $6281

O.1.   84 kg
        2.2 lb./kg = 185 lb./x
        x = 84 kg

O.2.   252 mg
        3 mg/kg = x/84 kg
        x = 252 mg

P.   *°C = 5/9 (°F – 32) = 5/9 (–90) = –50*

Q.   *°F = 32 + 9/5 °C = 32 + (–27) = 5*

Chapter Twelve

A.1. 3 tsp.
1 tsp./5 ml = x/15 ml

A.2. 6 tsp.
1 tsp./5 ml = x/30 ml
2 tbsp.
1 tbsp./15 ml = x/30 ml

A.3. 16 fluid oz.
480 ml
1 fluid oz./30 ml = 16 fluid oz./x
32 tbsp.
1 tbsp./15 ml = x/480 ml
96 tsp.
1 tbsp./3 tsp. = 32 tbsp./x
or
1 tsp./5 ml = x/480 ml

B.1. 2.2 lb.
454 g/1 lb. = 1000 g/x

B.2. 0.4 g
20 mg/2.2 lb. = x/44 lb.
x = 400 mg = 0.4 g

B.3. 133 mg
400 mg/3 doses = 133 mg/1 dose

B.4. approximately 1 tsp.
125 mg/1 tsp. = 133 mg/x
x = 1.064 tsp.

B.5. approximately 3 tsp.
125 mg/1 tsp. = 400 mg/x
x = 3.2 tsp.

B.6. 150 ml
15 ml/1 day = x/10 days

B.7. 5 fluid oz.
1 fluid oz./30 ml = x/150 ml

B.8. 21 doses
3 doses/1 day = x/7 days

C. 180 ml
Step 1: 15 ml/1 dose = x/4 doses
x = 60 ml/day
Step 2: 60 ml/1 day = x/3 days
x = 180 ml

D.1. 600 ml
Step 1: 30 drops/1 min. = x/360 min.
x = 10,800 drops
Step 2: 18 drops/1 ml = 10,800 drops/x
x = 600 ml

D.2. 5.4 g
0.9 g NaCl/100 ml = x/600 ml

E.1. 4.3 minutes
Step 1: 1 kg/2.2 lb.= 90 kg/x
x = 198 lb.
Step 2: 1 mcg/1 lb. = x/198 lb.
x = 198 mcg = 0.198 mg/min.
Step 3: 0.198 mg/1 min. = 0.85 mg/x
x = 4.3 minutes

E.2. 0.5 ml/min.
2 mg/5 ml = 0.198 mg/x
x = 0.5 ml/min.

E.3. 2.15 ml
0.5 ml/1 min. = x/4.3 min.
or
2 mg/5 ml = 0.85 mg/x
x = 2.13 ml

F. 3.33 ml
Step 1: 6 mg/lb. = x/50 lb.
x = 300 mg
Step 2: 90 mg/1 ml = 300 mg/x
x = 3.33 ml

G. 120 tablets
Step 1: 5 mg/lb. = x/100 lb.
x = 500 mg daily
Step 2: 125 mg/tab. = 500 mg/x
x = 4 tablets daily
Step 3: 4 tab./day = x/30 days
x = 120 tablets

H. 2.4 ml
Step 1: 1 kg/2.2 lb. = x/66 lb.
x = 30 kg patient's weight
Step 2: 10 mg/1 kg = x/30 kg
x = 300 mg
Step 3: 125 mg/1 ml = 300 mg/x
x = 2.4 ml

I. 0.4 ml
Step 1: 100 mcg = 0.1 mg
Step 2: 0.5 mg/2 ml = 0.1 mg/x
x = 0.4 ml

J. 0.59 mg
Step 1: 28 gtt./1 ml = 15 gtt./x
x = 0.54 ml
Step 2: 1.1 mg/1 ml = x/0.54 ml
x = 0.59 mg

K.   0.21 g
       30 mg/1 day = x/7 days
       x = 210 mg = 0.21 g

L.1.   36 tsp. doses
       1 tsp./5 ml = x/180 ml
       x = 36 tsp. doses

L.2.   6 days
       1 dose/4 hr. = 36 doses/x
       x = 144 hours = 6 days

M.   5 ml
       50 mcg/ml = 250 mcg/x
       x = 5 ml

N.1.   40 capsules
       1 × 4 × 10 = 40 capsules

N.2. $0.42
       40 cap./$16.80 = 1 cap./x
       x = $0.42

O.1.   150 ml
       5 ml × 3 × 10 = 150 ml

O.2.   10 days
       7.5 × 2 = 15 ml/day
       150 ml/15 ml = 10 days

P.1.   36 mg
       3 mg/1 lb. = x/12 lb.
       x = 36 mg

P.2.   4.5 ml
       8 mg/1 ml = 36 mg/x
       x = 4.5 ml

Q.1.   32 doses
       1 dose/15 ml = x/480 ml
       x = 32 doses

Q.2.   1.5 g
       10 g/100 ml = x/15 ml
       x = 1.5 g

Q.3.   48,000 mg
       10 g/100 ml = x/480 ml
       x = 48 g = 48,000 mg

R1.   125 ml
       1000 ml/8 hr. = x/1 hr.
       x = 125 ml

R.2.   21 gtt./min.
       125 ml/60 min. = x/1 min.
       x = 2.08 ml/min.
       10 gtt./1 ml = x/2.08 ml
       x = 21 gtt./min.

S.1.   1.8 m²
       Use adult nomogram to get 1.8 m²

S.2.   0.72 mg
       0.4 mg/1 m² = x/1.8 m²
       x = 0.72 mg

Chapter Thirteen

A.1.   19.2 g
       5 g triet./1000 ml = x/3840 ml
       x = 19.2 g = 19,200 mg
       1 g/1000 mg = 19.2 g/x

A.2.   148 gr.
       Step 1: 20 g/1000 ml = x/480 ml
       x = 9.6 g
       Step 2: 1 g/15.4 gr. = 9.6 g/x
       x = 148 gr.

A.3.   5 tsp.
       Step 1: 250 ml B.B./1000 ml lotion
       = x/100 ml lotion
       x = 25 ml B.B.
       Step 2: 1 tsp./5 ml = x/25 ml
       x = 5 tsp.

B.1.   1.67%
       2 g/120 g = 0.0167 = 1.67%

B.2.   16.7 mg
       2 g sulfur/120 g ung. = x/1 g ung.
       x = 0.0167 g = 1 6.7 mg

C.   4.4%
       20 g/454 g = 0.044 = 4.4%

D.1.   29.4%
       50 g/(50 g + 120 g) = 0.294 = 29.4%
       Note: The 50 g sulfur was added to
       120 g petrolatum, so the final
       product weighed 170 g.

D.2.   70.6%
       120 g pet./170 g ung. = 0.706 = 70.6%
       Note: One could also take previous answer and
       subtract from 100% (i.e., 100% – 29.4% = 70.6%).

E.   22.5 g ZnO
       0.25 × 90 g = 22.5 g

F.1.   6.25%
       30 ml/480 ml = 0.0625 = 6.25%

F.2. 3.75 ml
30 ml/480 ml = x/60 ml
or
0.0625× 60 = 3.75 ml

G. 4.67%
7 g/150 ml = 0.0467 = 4.67%

H.1. 11.8%
454 g/3840 ml = 0.118 = 11.8%

H.2. 1:8.46
454 g/3840 ml = 1/x
x = 8.46
Note: The ratio is 1/8.46 or 1:8.46.

I.1. 48 g
0.10 × 480 = 48

I.2. 10%
Note: Percent is the same for any volume
of a percent solution.

J. 2%
1:50 = 1/50 = 0.02 = 2%
19.2 g
0.02 × 960 ml = 19.2 g

K.1. 60 mg
Step 1: 6% means 6 g/100 ml or 6000 mg/100 ml
Step 2: 6000 mg/100 ml = x/1 ml

K.2. 1:16.67
6% = 6 g/100 ml
6 g/100 ml = 1/x
x = 16.67
Note: The ratio is 1/16.67
or 1:16.67.

L. 0.83%
Step 1: 2000 mg = 2 g and
8 fluid oz. = 240 ml
Step 2: 2 g/240 ml = 0.0083 = 0.83%
1:120
2 g/240 ml = 1/x x = 120
8.33 mg
2000 mg/240 ml = x/1 ml

M.1. 1:120
6/720 = 1/x   x = 120
so 6:720 equals 1:120

M.2. 0.833%
6/720 = 0.00833 = 0.833%

N.1. 1.063%
(30 ml) (17%) = (480 ml) (x)

N.2. 1:94
1.063/100 = 1/x   x = 94

N.3. 10.63 mg
Step 1: 1.063 g/100 ml =
1063 mg/100 ml
Step 2: 1063 mg/100 ml = x/1 ml
x = 10.63 mg

N.4. 0.85 g
0.17 × 5 ml = 0.85

N.5. 4.25%
(5 ml) (17%) = (20 ml) (x)
x = 4.25%
Note: The final solution is 20 ml
(5 ml added to 15 ml).

N.6. 78.54 gr.
Step 1: 0.17 × 30 = 5.1 g
Step 2: 1 g/15.4 gr. = 5.1 g/x
x = 78.54 gr.

N.7. 78.54 gr.
Note: The benzalkonium chloride in the
initial 30 ml is all that will be in the final
480 ml. The 30 ml was diluted with a diluent
that does not contain any additional
benzalkonium chloride.

N.8. 1:2000
(100 ml) (0.5%) = (1000 ml) (x)
x = 0.05% = 0.0005 = 5/10,000 =
5:10,000 = 1:2000

N.9. 2.5 mg
Step 1: 5 g/10,000 ml
5000 mg/10,000 ml
Step 2: 5000 mg/10,000 ml = x/5ml
or
0.0005 (5 ml) = 0.0025 g = 2.5 mg

O.1. yes
(10% is between 5% and 20%)

O.2. 151 g of 20%
Alligation Alternate Method
Note: The total amount made of
10% is the sum of the parts:
5 parts + 10 parts = 15 parts
In this case, it is 454 g, so

$$\frac{15\ parts}{454\ g} = \frac{5\ parts}{x}$$

303 g of 5%
15 parts/454 = 10 parts/x
or 454 g (total) – 151 g (of 20%) = 303 g of 5%

O.3. 90 g of 10%
5 parts/30 g = 15 parts/x   x = 90 g

P.1. no
(10% is not between 20% and 15%)

P.2. not possible

P.3. not possible

Q. 9 g NaCl
0.009 × 1000 ml = 9 g
153.8 mEq Na⁺
58.5 mg/L mEq = 9000 mg/x
Note: MW of NaCl = 58.5.

R.1. 0.745%
Step 1: MW KCl = 74.5 mg = 1 mEq
Step 2: 10 mEq = 745 mg = 0.745 g
Step 3: 0.745 g/100 ml =
0.00745 = 0.745%

R.2. 7450 mg
Step 1: 10 mEq/100 ml =
x/1000 ml
x = 100 mEq
Step 2: 1 mEq KCl/74.5 mg
KCl = 100 mEq KCl/x
x = 7450 mg

S. 4.5 mEq
Step 1: mEq CaCl2 = 111/2= 55.5 mg
Step 2: 55.5 mg/1 mEq = 250 mg/x

T. 1.67%
Step 1: 250 mg = 0.25 g
Step 2: 0.25 g/15 ml =
0.0167 = 1.67%

U. 38.5 mEq
Step 1: MW of Al(OH)₃ = 78
Step 2: 1 mEq = 78/3 = 26 mg
Step 3: 1 mEq Al(OH)₃/26 mg =
x/1000 mg
x = 38.5 mEq

V.1. 200 ml
5 ml/dose × 4 doses/day ×
10 days = 200 ml

V.2. 40 ml
200 ml – 160 ml H₂O = 40 ml

V.3. 7 g
1 g/1 day = x/7 days
x = 7 g

W. 8.33 tablets
Step 1: 1 cap./5 mg codeine = 50 cap./x
x = 250 mg
Step 2: 30 mg/1 tab. = 250 mg/x
x = 8.33 tablets

X.1. 12 tablets
Step 1: (0.02 × 150) = 3 g = 3000 mg
Step 2: 250 mg/1 tab. = 3000 mg/x
x = 12 tablets

X.2. 1:50
Note: 1 tsp. of 2% is still 2%, so 2% = 0.02
= 2/100 = 2:100 = 1:50

X.3. 20 mg
Step 1: 2% × 150 = 3 g = 3000 mg
Step 2: 3000 mg/150 ml = x/1 ml
x = 20 mg

Y.1. 7500 mg
500 mg/1 ml =x/15
x = 7500 mg

Y.2. no

Y.3. yes

Y.4. 2.2 ml
15 ml (final volume) – 12.8 ml
(diluent) = 2.2 ml (powder volume displacement)

Y.5. 4 ml
500 mg/1 ml = 2000 mg/x
x = 4 ml

Y.6. 3.25 ml
10 ml (diluent) + 2.2 ml (powder
volume displacement) = 12.2 ml
(final volume containing 7500 mg of
the drug)
7500 mg/12.2 ml = 2000 mg/x
x = 3.25 ml

Z.1. 8.25%
Alligation Medial Method

0.5 kg	*×*	*3%*	*=*	*1.5 kg%*
1.5 kg	*×*	*10%*	*=*	*15.0 kg%*
2 kg				*16.5 kg%*

16.5kg%/2 kg = 8.25%

Z.2. 1:12.12
8.25/100 = 1/x
x = 12.12

Z.3. 37.5 g
454 × 8.25% = 37.5 g

151

Z.4.   no

Z.5.   *237.8 g*

Step 1: Alligation Alternate Method

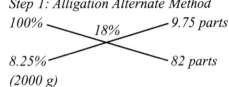

(2000 g)

Step 2: *82 parts/2000 g =*
9.75 parts/x
x = 237.8 g

Chapter Fourteen

A.1. $20
        1 cap./$0.20 = 100 cap./x
        x = $20
A.2. $0.25 each
        $0.20 cost plus $0.05 profit
A.3. $7.50
        1 cap./$0.25 = 30 cap./x
        x = $7.50
B.1. $10
        Selling Price = Cost + Markup
        $60 = $50 + Markup
        Markup = $60 – $50 = $10
B.2.   20%
        Markup/Cost = $10/$50 = 0.2 = 20%
B.3.   16.7%
        Markup/Selling price = $10/$60 = 0.167 = 16.7%
C.1. $20
        $65 – $45 = $20 markup
C.2.   31%
        $20/$65 = 0.31 = 31%
C.3.   44%
        $20/$45 = 0.44 = 44%
C.4. $77.40
        1.72 × $45 = $77.40
D.1. $55
        $65 – $10 = $55
D.2. $1.63
        40 cap./$65 = 1 cap./x
        x = $1.63/cap.

D.3. $0.25
        $10 markup/40 cap. = x/1 cap.
        x = $0.25
D.4. $22.75
        40 cap./$65 = 14 cap./x
        x = $22.75
D.5.   18%
        $10/$55 = 0.18 = 18%
D.6.   15.4%
        $10/$65 = 0.154 = 15.4%

Chapter Fifteen (Practice Questions)

1.   c
2.   d
        1 g/30,000 ml = x/3000
        x = 0.1 g = 100 mg
3.   b
        Step 1: 250 units/1 g = x/1000 g
        x = 250,000 units
        Step 2: 500 units/1 g =
        250,000 units/x   x = 500 g
4.   c
5.   a
        Step 1: 10,000 mcg = 10 mg= 0.01 g
        Step 2: 0.1 g/10 ml = 0.01 g/x
        x = 1 ml
6.   d
        0.25% × 30 = 0.0025 × 30 =
        0.075 g = 75 mg
7.   c
8.   c
        Step 1: 30 mEq/1000 ml = 5 mEq/x
        x = 167 ml
        Step 2: 167 ml/60 min. = x/1 min.
        x = 2.78 ml/min.
        Step 3: 15 gtt./1 ml = x/2.78 ml
        x = 41.7 or 42 gtt./min
9.   a
        0.9 g/100 ml = 60 g/x
        x = 6666 ml = 6.67 L

10.   d

Step 1: Alligation Alternate Method

5% → 12 parts
8%
20% → 3 parts

(180 g)

Step 2: 3 parts/180 g = 12 parts/x
x = 720 g

11.   b

2000 mg/5.8 ml = x/1 ml
x = 345 mg

12.   d

13.   b

14.   a

Step 1: 2.2 lb./1 kg = 220 lb./x
x = 100 kg
Step 2: 5 mcg/1 kg = x/100 kg
x = 500 mcg = 0.5 mg/min.
Step 3: 0.5 mg/1 min = x/60 min.
x = 30 mg per hour
Step 4: 800 mg/500 ml = 30 mg/x
x = 18.75 ml
Note: Sometimes μg is used to represent
micrograms or mcg.

15.   c

Step 1: 2.2 lb./1 kg = 264 lb./x
x = 120 kg
Step 2: 10 mg/1 kg = x/120 kg
x = 1200 mg
Step 3: 200 mg/1 tab. = 1200 mg/x
x = 6 tab.

16.   c

1 g/750 ml = x/960 ml
x = 1.28 g

17.   c

18.   a

Step 1: total weight of recipe:
400 + 150 + 100 + 350 = 1000 g
Step 2: 400 g glycerin/1000 g
zinc gel = x/454 g zinc gel
x = 181.6 g

19.   d

20.   b

Step 1: 1/2 pt. = 240 ml
Step 2: 2 gal. = 7680 ml
Step 3: 1 bottle/240 ml = x/7680ml
x = 32 bottles

21.   b

22.   b

Step 1: Alligation Medial Method
  90 ml × 14% = 1260 ml%
  100 ml × 0% = 0
  40 ml × 78% = 3120 ml%

230 ml   4380 ml%
Step 2: 4380 ml%/230 ml = 19.04%

23.   c

24.   c

Step 1: 2.2 lb./1 kg = 38 lb./x
x = 17.27 kg
Step 2: 35 mg/1 kg = x/17.27 kg
x = 604.54 mg (total daily dose)
Step 3: 604.54 mg/6 doses =
x/1 dose
x = 100.8 mg per dose

25.   d

0.5 mg/2 ml = x/0.75 ml
x = 0.1875 mg = 187.5 mcg

26.   a

27.   a

Step 1: 1 mEq = 74.5 mg/L
(valence) = 74.5 mg
Step 2: 74.5 mg/1 mEq = x/3 mEq
x = 223.5 mg
Step 3: 223.5 mg/5 ml = x/1000 ml
x = 44,700 mg = 44.7 g

28.   a

(old vol.)(old %) = (new vol.)(new %)
(O.V.)(0%) = (N.V.)(N.%)
(x) (20%) = (600 ml) (0.5%)
x = 15 ml

29.   b

30. b

Step 1: Alligation Alternate Method

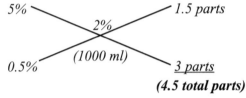

1%

(30 g)   5%   95 parts

100%   4 parts

Step 2: 95 parts/30 g = 4 parts/x

x = 1.26 g

31. c

500 mcg/15 ml = x/1000 ml

x = 33,333 mcg= 33.33 mg

32. c

3 g/$24.50 = 0.5 g/x

x= $4.08

33. d

Step 1: 500 mg/1 dose = x/4 doses

x = 2000 mg/day

Step 2: 2000 mg/1 day = x/10 days

x = 20,000 mg for 10 days

Step 3: 250 mg/5 ml = 20,000 mg/x

x = 400 ml

34. c

35. d

36. d

Step 1: Alligation Alternate Method

95%   10 parts

          40%

30%   (2000 ml)   55 parts

                    (65 total parts)

Step 2: 65 parts/2000 ml = 10 parts/x

x = 308 ml

37. a

Step 1: 4 × 480 ml = 1920 ml

Step 2: 1 g/1000 ml = x/1920 ml

x = 1.92 g

38. b

Step 1: 1 mEq potassium gluconate =

MW/valence = 234/1 = 234 mg

Step 2: 2 tbsp. = 30 ml

Step 3: 30 ml × 30% = 9 g

(i.e., 30 ml × 0.3 = 9 g)

Step 4: 9 g = 9000 mg

Step 5: 1 mEq potassium gluconate/

234 mg = x/9000 mg

x = 38.46 mEq

39. b

180 mg/5 ml = 280 mg/x

x = 7.78 ml

40. d

(Examples include oral contraceptives, products containing estrogenic or progestational agents, isotretinoin, intrauterine devices, and isoproterenol inhalation devices.)

41. b

42. d

Step 1: Alligation Alternate Method

5%   1.5 parts

          2%

0.5%   (1000 ml)   3 parts

                    (4.5 total parts)

Step 2: 4.5 parts/1000 ml = 3 parts/x

x = 667 ml

43. b

Step 1: 18 g/1000 ml = x/5 ml

x = 0.09 g = 90 mg

Step 2: 65 mg/1 gr. = 90 mg/x

x = 1.38 gr.

44. c

Step 1: 1 g/15.4 gr. = 28 g/x

x = 431.2 gr.

Step 2: 13/8 gr./1 cap. =

431.2 gr./x

x = 313 capsules

45. b

$8.75/120 ml = x/15 ml

x = $1.09

46. a

Step 1: 1 mEq = MW/valence =

389/1 = 389 mg

Step 2: 1 mEq K. pcn. V/389 mg =

x/2000 mg

x = 5.14 mEq

47. a

Step 1: 1200 mg/60 min. = x/1 min.

x = 20 mg/min.

Step 2: 50 mg/1 ml = 20 mg/x

x = 0.4 ml

48.　b

Step 1: 2.2 lb./1 kg = 5.5 lb./x
x = 2.5 kg (infant's weight)
Step 2: 2.5 mg gentamicin/
1 kg = x/2.5 kg
x = 6.25 mg (dose)
Step 3: 20 mg gentamicin/1 ml =
6.25 mg gentamicin/x
x = 0.31 ml

49.　c

Step 1: 1 mEq calcium =
AW/valence = 40/2 = 20 mg
Step 2: 1 mEq/20 mg = 5 mEq/x
x = 100 mg
Step 3: 100 mg/50 ml = x/1000 ml
x = 2000 mg/L

50.　d

2% × 60 g = 1.2 g = 1200 mg
benzocaine
(i.e., 0.02 × 60 = 1.2)

51.　d

Step 1: 400 gr. × 3/8 = 150 gr.
Step 2: 437.5 gr. – 150 gr.= 287.5 gr.

52.　c

53.　d

1000 mg/4.1 ml = 675 mg/x
x = 2.77 ml

54.　c

Step 1: From problem #53 the dry powder
displacement is 0.7 ml
4.1 – 3.4 = 0.7 ml
Step 2: For problem #54
4.3 ml + 0.7 ml = 5 ml
(new and incorrect volume)
Step 3: Note: the 5 ml contains 1 g of nafcillin
1000 mg/5 ml = 675 mg/x
x = 3.375 = 3.4 ml

55.　b

Step 1: 0.1% = 0.1 g/100 ml =
100 mg/100 ml
Step 2: 100 mg/100 ml = 75 mg/x
x = 75 ml

56.　c

°F = 32 + 9/5 °C
°F = 32 + (9/5 × 65)
°F = 32 + 117
°F = 149

57.　b

58.　d

Step 1: 50% = 50 g/100 ml
Step 2: 50 g/100 ml = x/1000 ml
x = 500 g
Step 3: 1 g dextrose/3.4 cal =
500 g dextrose/x
x = 1700 calories

59.　b

2 g coal tar/60 g formula =
x/454 g formula
x = 15.1 g coal tar

60.　b

Step 1: 1000 units/60 min. = x/1 min.
x = 16.67 units per minute
Step 2: 20,000 units/500 ml =
16.67 units/x
x = 0.42 ml per minute
Step 3: 15 gtt./1 ml = x/0.42 ml
x = 6.3 gtt. = 6 gtt./min.

61.　d

Step 1: 40 g = 40,000 mg =
40,000,000 mcg
Step 2: 600 mcg/1 tab. =
40,000,000 mcg/x
x = 66,666 tablets

62.　d

*Note: Since the diluent is **zero***
percent, this problem can be worked
several ways. The easiest method is
by a simple dilution, i.e., (old volume)
(old %) = (new volume)(new %).
A second method is alligation alternate,
but it requires additional work.

(O.V.) (O.%) = (N.V.) (N.%)
(454 g) (20%) = (x) (5%)
x = 1816 g of 5%

63.　c

Step 1: 0.25% = 0.25 g/100 ml =
250 mg/100 ml
Step 2: 250 mg/100 ml = x/15 ml
x = 37.5 mg
or
0.25% × 15 ml = 0.0375 g = 37.5 mg

64.   a
      Step 1: 5000 ml × 0.9% =
      5000 × 0.009 = 45 g
      Step 2: 2.25 g/1 tab. = 45 g/x
      x = 20 tablets

65.   c
      Step 1: Total parts in this formula
      equal 15
      1 + 6 + 8 = 15 parts
      Step 2: 15 parts powder/1000 g =
      6 parts/x
      x = 400 g of calcium carbonate

66.   c
      Step 1: 5 mg/1 ml = 2.5 mg/x
      x = 0.5 ml per dose
      Step 2: 0.5 ml/1 dose = 10 ml/x
      x = 20 doses

67.   c
      *Note: Diluent is **zero** percent*
      so this can be solved by 2 methods.
      Step 1: (O.V.) (O.%) = (N.V.) (N.%)
      (960 ml) (10%) = (x) (3%)
      x = 3200 ml of 3% dilution made,
      but how much water must be added
      to the 960 ml?
      Step 2: 3200 ml – 960 ml =
      2240 ml of water added
      or
      Step 1: Alligation Alternate Method

      10%   *3 parts*
      (960 ml)   *3%*

      0%   *7 parts*

      Step 2: 3 parts/960 ml = 7 parts/x
      x = 2240 ml water

68.   c

69.   a
      10 lb. = 4540 g = 4.54 kg
      4.54 kg/340,000 tab. = x/170,000 tab.
      x = 2.27 kg

70.   b

71.   a
      50 mg/15 ml = x/960 ml
      x = 3200 mg = 3.2 g

72.   b
      0.25 mg/1 tab. = x/50 tab.
      x = 12.5 mg
      65 mg/1gr. = 12.5 mg/x
      x = 0.192 gr.

73.   a

74.   b
      80 mg/2 ml = 20 mg/x
      x = 0.5 ml

75.   c
      18 gtt./1 ml = x/500 ml
      x = 9000 gtt.

76.   b

77.   a
      30 mg/1 m² = x/0.7 m²
      x = 21 mg

78.   d
      1 × 2 × 90 = 180

79.   b
      500 mcg/ml = 250 mcg/x
      x = 0.5 ml

80.   b
      46/2.2 = 21 kg
      4 mg/1 kg = x/21 kg
      x = 84 mg

81.   d
      2 × 2 × 90 = 360

82.   a
      0.2 mg/15 ml = x/480 ml
      x = 6.4 mg

83.   b
      8.8/2.2 = 4 kg
      2.5 mg/1 kg = x/4 kg
      x = 10 mg b.i.d. = 20 mg daily

84.   d

85.   a
      1000 ml/480 min. = x/1 min.
      x = 2.08 ml

86.   a
      12.5 mg/5 ml = x/960 ml
      x = 2400 mg = 2.4 g

87.   a

88.   a
      150 g/1000 tab. = x/50,000
      x = 7500 g = 7.5 kg

89. d

   250 g/1000 tab. = 2270 g/x

   x = 9080 tablets

90. c

   total weight of formula is 525.75 g

   0.75/525.75 = 0.00143 = 0.143%

91. b

   10 ml – 7.8 ml = 2.2 ml

92. b

   100 mg/1 ml = 300 mg/x

   x = 3 ml

93. a

   100 mg/1 ml = x/10 ml

   x = 1000 mg = 1 g

94. b

   250 × 4 × 10 = 10,000 mg

   1 g/1 vial = 10 g/x   x = 10 vials

95. b

   2.2 + 9.8 = 12 ml per vial and it still

   contains 1000 mg of drug

   1000 mg/12 ml = 250 mg/x

   x = 3 ml

96. c

   1000 ml/12 hr. = x/1 hr.

   x = 83.3 ml

97. d

   4,000,000 units/720 min. = x/1 min.

   x = 5555 units

98. a

   1000 ml/720 min. = x/1 min.

   x = 1.39 ml/min.

99. d

   1000 ml/12 hr. = x/1 hr.

   x = 83.3 ml

   15 gtt./1 ml = x/83.3 ml

   x = 1250 gtt.

100. d

   1 g benz./500 g oint. = x/120 g oint.

   x = 0.24 g = 240 mg

101. c

   5 g pre. sulf./100 g oint. = x/1000 g oint.

   x = 50 g

102. c

103. b

   Alligation Medial Method

1 kg	×	10%	=	10 kg%
+ 1 kg	×	15%	=	15 kg%
+ 1 kg	×	20%	=	20 kg%

   3 kg   45 kg%

   45 kg%/3 kg = 15%

104. c

   (O.V.) (O.%) = (N.V.) (N.%)

   (30 ml) (20%) = (1000 ml) (x)

   x = 0.6%

105. d

   0.6/100 = 1/x

   x = 167 = 1:167

106. d

   0.6 g/100 ml = x/15 ml

   x = 0.09 g = 90 mg

107. c

108. d

   Note: Using the alligation alternate

   technique, you will need 10 parts of

   95% alcohol and 40 parts of 45%

   alcohol to make 50 parts of 55% alcohol.

109. b

   50 parts/1000 ml = 10 parts/x

   x = 200 ml of 95%

110. d

   50 parts/1000 ml = 40 parts/x

   x = 800 ml of 45%

111. b

   10 parts/480 ml = 50 parts/x

   x = 2400 ml of 55%

112. b

113. c

   $14.88/12 = $1.24 (cost per tube)

   $2.69 – $1.24 = $1.45 markup

114. c

   $1.45/$2.69 = 0.54 = 54%

115. d

   $1.45/$1.24 = 1.17 = 117%

116. c

   $2.69 × 0.7 = $1.88

117. c

118. b

119. d

120. c

Answer Key

121.   c
       Alendronate is the generic name for Fosamax®.
       Actonel® is available in a formulation with
       calcium, whereas Fosamax® is available in
       a formulation with vitamin D.

122.   c
       1200 cal/1000 ml = x/1500 ml
       x = 1800 calories

123.   d
       43 g/1000 ml = x/60 ml
       x = 2.6 g = 2600 mg

124.   a
       39 + 170 = 209 g/bottle
       209 g/1 bottle = x/2 bottles
       x = 418 g = 0.418 kg

125.   d
       2000 mg/1000 ml = 160 mg/x
       x = 80 ml/hr.

126.   d
       10 g/1000 ml = x/15 ml
       x = 0.15 g = 150 mg = 150,000 mcg

Appendix A

Common Dosage Forms

aerosol	lozenge
capsule	ointment
cream	paste
drops	patch
elixir	pellet or implant
emulsion	powder
enema	solution
extract	suppository
gel	suspension
granule	syrup
injection	tablet
lotion	tincture

Drug Administration Routes

buccal	oral
epidural	otic
inhalation	parenteral
intra-arterial	perivascular
intracardiac	rectal
intramuscular	subcutaneous
intranasal	sublingual
intraperitoneal	topical
intrathecal	transdermal
intravenous	urethral
nasal	urogenital
ophthalmic	vaginal

Appendix B

Common Abbreviations Used in Prescriptions and Medication Orders

a	before	GI	gastrointestinal
a.a. or aa	of each	gr.	grain
a.c.	before meals	gtt.	drop
ad	up to	h. or hr.	hour
a.d.	right ear	h.s.	at bedtime
ad lib.	at pleasure	hx	history
a.m.	morning	H_2O	water
ante	before	IM	intramuscular
aq.	aqueous (water)	inj.	injection
a.s.	left ear	IV	intravenous
a.u.	each ear	IVP	intravenous push
b.i.d.	twice a day	IVPB	intravenous piggyback
c. or c	with	K	potassium
cap.	capsule	KCl	potassium chloride
cc.	cubic centimeter (milliliter)	L or l	liter
Cl	chloride	lb.	pound
comp.	compound	LR	lactated Ringer's
D.A.W.	dispense as written	mcg or µg	microgram
D.C., dc, or disc.	discontinue	mEq	milliequivalent
dil.	dilute	Mg	magnesium
disp.	dispense	mg	milligram
div.	divide	min.	minute
d.t.d.	give of such doses	ml	milliliter
dx	diagnosis	Na	sodium
D5NS	5% dextrose in 0.9% sodium chloride	NaCl	sodium chloride
D5RL	5% dextrose in Ringer's lactate	N.F.	National Formulary
		noct.	night
D5W	5% dextrose in water	non rep.	do not repeat
elix.	elixir	NPO	nothing by mouth
et	and	NR	no refill
ex. aq.	in water	NS	normal saline (0.9% sodium chloride)
ft.	make	NTG	nitroglycerin
g or gm or Gm	gram	N/V	nausea and/or vomiting
gal.	gallon	o.d.	right eye

o.l. or o.s.	left eye	rt., R	right
o.u.	both eyes	s. or $\bar{s}$	without
oz.	ounce	sec.	second
p	after	Sig.	write on label
p.c.	after meals	SL, sl	sublingual
p.m.	afternoon; evening	sol.	solution
p.o.	by mouth	ss. or $\bar{s}\,\bar{s}$	one half
pr	per rectum	SSKI	saturated solution of
p.r.n.	as needed		potassium iodide
pt.	pint	stat	immediately
pulv.	powder	s.c. or s.q.	subcutaneously
q.	every	supp.	suppository
q.d.	every day	susp.	suspension
q.h.	every hour	syr.	syrup
q.h.s.	every bedtime	tab.	tablet
q.i.d.	four times a day	tbsp. or T	tablespoonful
q.o.d.	every other day	t.i.d.	three times a day
q.s.	a sufficient quantity	TPN	total parenteral nutrition
q.s. ad	a sufficient quantity	tr. or tinct.	tincture
	to make	tsp. or t.	teaspoonful
qt.	quart	u.d.	as directed
RL	Ringer's lactate	ung.	ointment
R/O	rule out	U.S.P.	United States Pharmacopoeia

Notes:

Notes:

Notes:

Notes:

Notes:

Notes:

Notes:

Notes: